Gastric Revision Operations

Single Surgical Procedures 33

A Colour Atlas of

Gastric Revision Operations

John Alexander-Williams

MD, ChM, FRCS, FACS

Consultant Surgeon,
The General Hospital, Birmingham.
Honorary Clinical Senior Lecturer,
University of Birmingham.
Formerly External Scientific Staff Medical Research Council.
Formerly Hunterian Professor Royal College of Surgeons of England.

Photography by Gareth J. Hyland
TEC Diploma in Medical Photography
Senior Medical Photographer
General and Dental Hospitals, Birmingham

Wolfe Medical Publications Ltd

Year Book Medical Publishers, Inc

Published by Wolf Medical Publications Ltd, 1986
Printed by W.S. Cowell Ltd, 8 Buttermarket, Ipswich
United Kingdom
ISBN 0 7234 1055 0

This book is one of the titles in the series of Wolfe Single Surgical Procedures, a series which will eventually cover some 200 titles.

For a full list of Atlases in this series, plus forthcoming titles and details of our surgical, dental and veterinary Atlases, please write to Wolfe Medical Publications Ltd, Wolfe House, 3 Conway Street, London W1P 6HE
or
Year Book Medical Publishers, Inc, 35 East Wacker Drive, Chicago, Ill. 60601

Distributed in Continental North and Central America, Hawaii and Puerto Rico by Year Book Medical Publishers, Inc.

Library of Congress Cataloging in Publication Data

Alexander-Williams, John.
Color atlas of gastric revision operations.

(Single surgical procedures series ; v. 33)
Spine title: Gastric revision operations.
1. Peptic ulcer—Surgery—Complications and sequelae—Atlases. 2. Stomach—Surgery—Atlases. I. Title. II. Title: Gastric revision operations. III. Series.
[DNLM: 1. Stomach—surgery—atlases.
WI 17 A379c]
RD540.53.A44 1986 617'.5541 85-8901
ISBN 0-87489-538-3

We list below a few of the other titles in print and in preparation in the Single Surgical Procedures series. For a comprehensive list please write.

Published
Parotidectomy
Traditional Meniscectomy
Inguinal Hernias & Hydroceles in Infants and Children
Surgery for Pancreatic & Associated Carcinomata
Subtotal Thyroidectomy
Anterior Resection of Rectum
Boari Bladder-Flap Procedure
Surgery for Varicose Veins
Treatment of Carpal Tunnel Syndrome
Seromyotomy for Chronic Duodenal Ulcer
Surgery for Undescended Testes
Operations on the Internal Carotid Artery
Renal Transplant
Lumbar Discography
Visceral Artery Reconstruction
Flexor Tendon Repair
Proctocolectomy
Common Operations of the Foot
Right Hemicolectomy
Extra-cranial and Intra-cranial Anastomosis
Surgery for Hirschsprung's Disease
Thyroid Lobectomy
Surgery at the Thoracic Outlet
External Fixation
Anterior Cervical Spine Fusion
Liver Transplantation
Modified Radical Mastectomy
Paratopic Transplant of Body and Tail of the Pancreas
Subdiaphragmatic Total Gastrectomy for Malignant Disease
Rupture of the Rotator Cuff
Left Hemicolectomy

In Production
Surgery of Lymphoedema of the Lower Limbs
Gastric Revision Operations
Plastering Techinques
Cleft Lip Surgery
Mastectomy with Immediate Reconstruction
Joint Replacement of the Hand
Periodontal Surgery

Some Future Titles
Biliary Enteric Anastomosis with Strictures in Common Bile Duct
Surgical Disencumberment of the Thoracic Outlet
Aortic Endarterectomy
Axillary Dissection for Melanoma
Groin Dissection for Melanoma
Coronary Artery Bypass
Omental Transposition
Orthopaedic Hip Approaches
Management of Venous Disease
Upper Thoracic Sympathectomy
Inguinal Hernia Repair
Vascular Access
Dental Analgesia
Hiatus Hernia
Plastic and Reconstructive Surgery
Occlusion/Malocclusion
Femoral and Tibial Osteotomy
Resection of Aortic Aneurysm
Ileo-Rectal Anastomosis
Techniques of Nerve Grafting and Repair
Surgery for Dupuytren's Contracture
Athrodesis of the Ankle
Spondylolisthesis
Repair of Prolapsed Rectum
Splenectomy
Anterior Nephrectomy
Caecocystoplasty
Total Gastrectomy
Billroth 1 Gastrectomy
Billroth 2 Gastrectomy
Abdominal Incisions
Thoracotomy
Appendicectomy
Incisional Hernia
Lung Lobectomy
Lung Removal
Haemorrhoids
Rectosigmoid Resection
Surgery for Anorectal Incontinence
Visceral Vascular Occlusion
Aortofemoral Bypass
Aortoilac Disobliteration
Joint Replacement of Wrist and Hand
Operative Fixation of Fractures of the Forearm
Minor Operative Procedures
Technique of Arthroscopy of the Knee

Contents

Introduction

Operation for the permanent cure for gastric and duodenal ulceration usually involved vagotomy of partial gastric resection or both; they have a low mortality and are usually successful in curing the ulcer. Generally, operations that disturb physiology the least, such as proximal gastric or highly selective vagotomy have the highest rate of recurrent ulcer. Whereas, the more major operations such as vagotomy and antrectomy or subtotal gastric resection have the lowest risk of recurrent ulcer but the highest risk of producing new symptoms as a result of the altered physiology.

Since the advent of effective ulcer-curing drugs with few side-effects such as cimetedine and ranitidine, there have been three changes of emphasis in the selection of patients for ulcer curative surgery. First, less patients have been submitted for surgical treatment and second, because the complication of recurrent ulceration can usually be managed quite readily by histamine H_2 receptor blockade, surgeons are becoming less obsessed by the risk of recurrence and more concerned about the risk of inducing other less easily managed postgastric operation problems. The third change is that the decreased number of ulcer curative operations has meant that surgeons in training, or in relatively small communities have difficulty in maintaining the high degree of technical expertise necessary to perfect such complicated operations as proximal gastric vagotomy, which are now tending to be performed only in highly specialised and interested centres.

In my own practice the need for gastric revisions for failed ulcer curative operations has decreased. Twenty to 30 years ago there was a change from gastric resection to vagotomy. However, it still remains true that about 80 per cent of patients having ulcer curative surgery are pleased with the results, whereas 20 per cent or more continue to have symptoms sufficiently severe to warrant treatment. It is in this group of patients that remedial gastric surgery can be considered as one of the options of treatment.

We recognise several distinct facets of the postgastrectomy and postvagotomy syndrome such as dumping, gastric retention, bile vomiting, diarrhoea, as well as recurrent ulceration. Although these syndromes can often be separated clinically and accurately categorized with the aid of both simple and sophisticated measurements, most patients exhibit a combined symptom pattern, that includes some aspects of one syndrome and some aspects of another. It is rarely, if ever, possible to categorize a patient into one pure symptom group. Therefore, in the evaluation of these patients it is necessary to assess all aspects of the various problems that can occur as a result of the altered physiology brought about by operations designed to cure chronic peptic ulceration.

This book does not aim to discuss in detail the methods of assessment but I would be wrong if I were to tell any surgical colleague how I do a particular operation without emphasizing that I only do it after the most exhaustive assessment that requires the facilities of a well-equipped and research orientated gastroenterology unit. I will refer here simply to the broad categories of tests that should be or could be performed before operation.

Investigative procedures

1

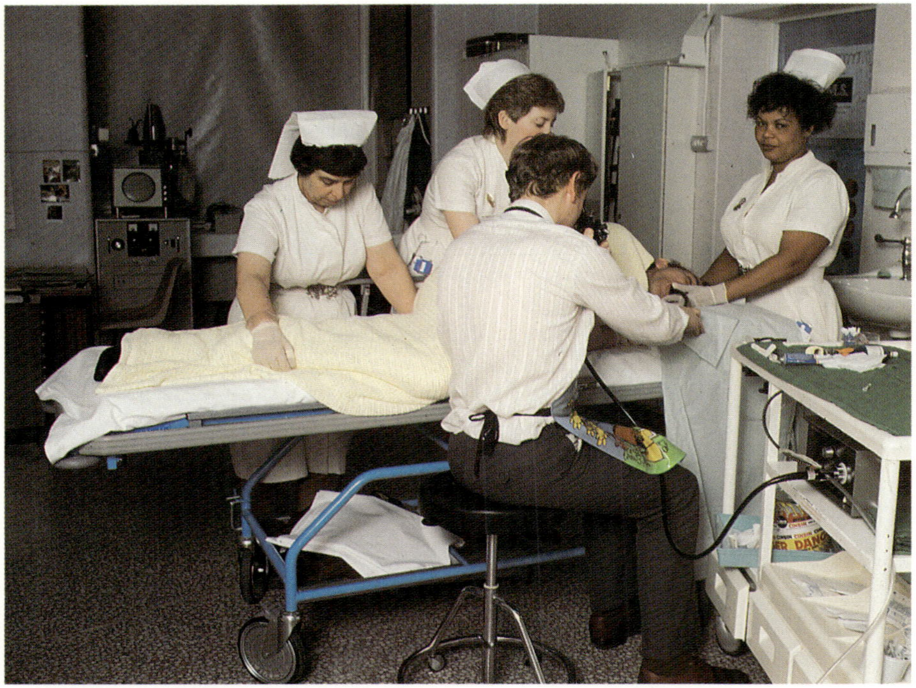

1 **Fibreoptic endoscopy of the upper gastrointestinal tract** is the most important method of investigating the patient who still has dyspeptic symptoms after an operation designed to cure peptic ulceration.

2

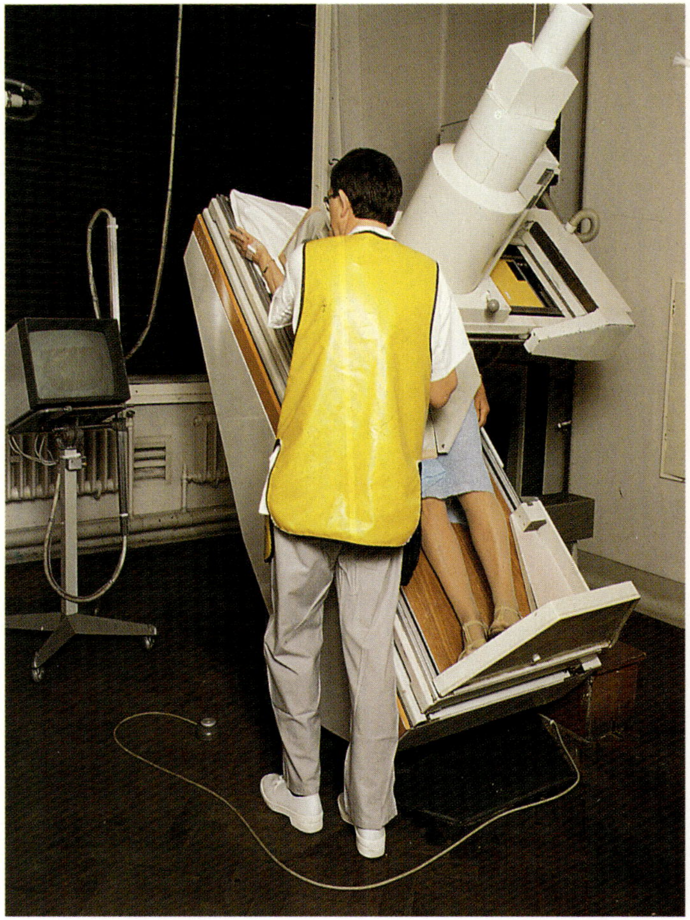

2 **Barium meal examination is less informative than endoscopy** but it is still necessary to show the anatomy of the stomach or gastric remnant. Oral cholecystogram and/or ultrasound examination of the gall bladder are advisable to complete the diagnostic work-up.

3

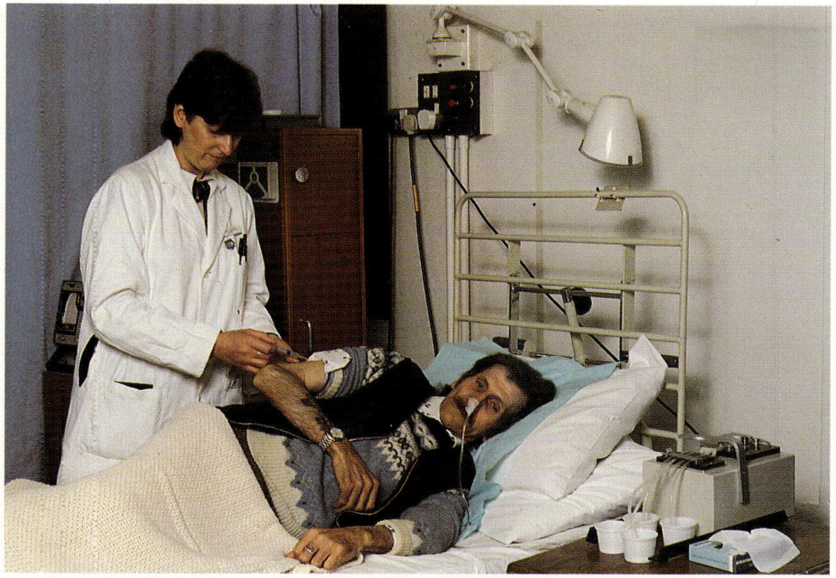

3 Acid secretory studies are an essential part of the investigation of patients after gastric operations. After an overnight fast the patient has a double lumen airbleed, nasogastric tube inserted. The patient lies on the left side in the semi-recumbent position. We do not use xray screening of the tube but check that it is in the stomach by the water recovery test. After a half hour collection of basal secretion, the patient receives 0.5 mg per kilogram of Pentogastrin subcutaneously and quarter hourly samples are collected for estimations of free hydrochloric acid and pH.

The aspiration test can also be used to measure free bile acids and to culture the gastric contents. The latter will allow appropriate peroperative antibiotic prophylaxis to be given, if surgical treatment has to be undertaken.

The insulin hypoglycaemia test is also used in some centres to test the completeness of vagotomy but we do not do this routinely. **The insulin test is unpleasant and sometimes dangerous.** If the patient requires an operation, we prefer an intraoperative elective test of vagal innervation (see below).

4

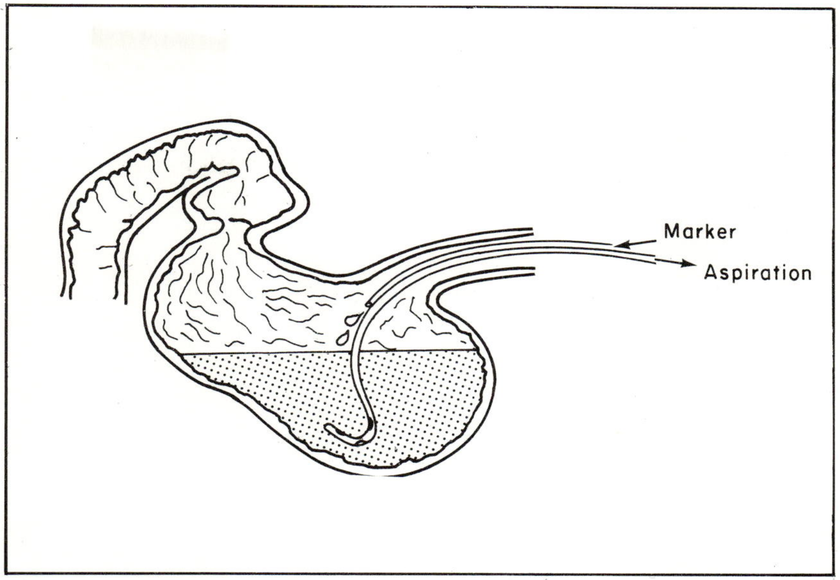

4 Diagrammatic representation of the nasogastric tube lying within the body of the stomach with the patient in the left lateral position. Some workers advise checking on the rate of recovery of gastric contents by instilling a detectable marker such as Polyethylene glycol or Phenol red.

5 As a measure of reflux and bile into the stomach or the oesophagus we use the technetium labelled synthetic bile salt derivative HIDA, as the patient lies prone under a 90cm field of view gamma camera for 90 minutes.

5

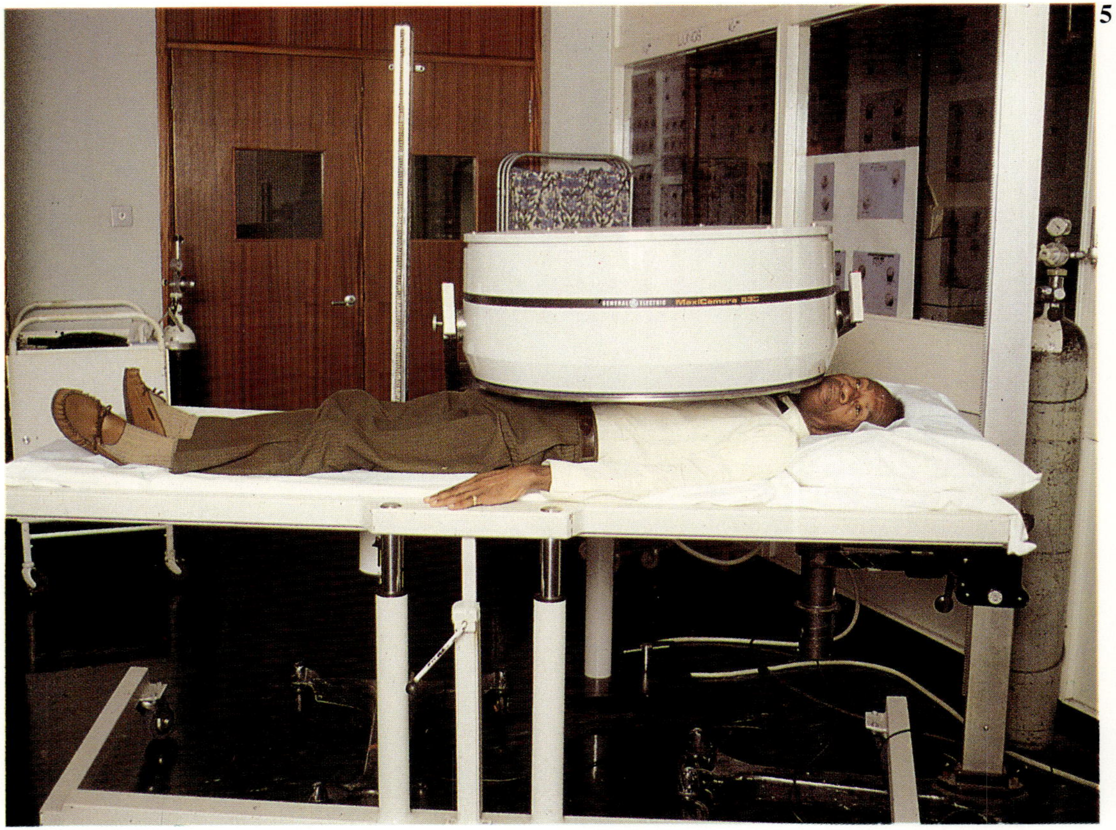

6

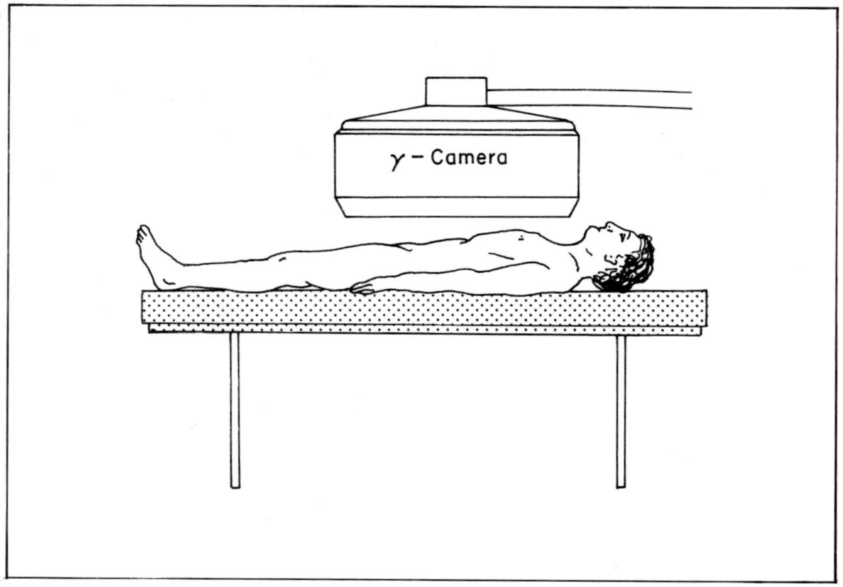

6 **Patient having isotope scan for bile reflux lying prone beneath a 90 cm field of view gamma camera.**

7

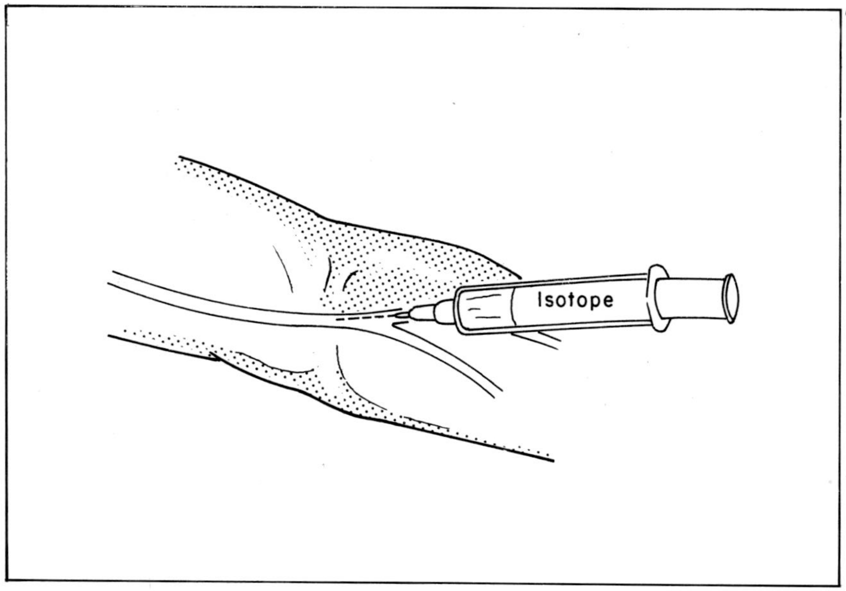

7 **HIDA is injected intravenously.**

8 The data from the gamma camera are fed into a computer that uses correction formulae to allow for degradation of the radioisotope and radioactive scatter from without and within the area of interest.

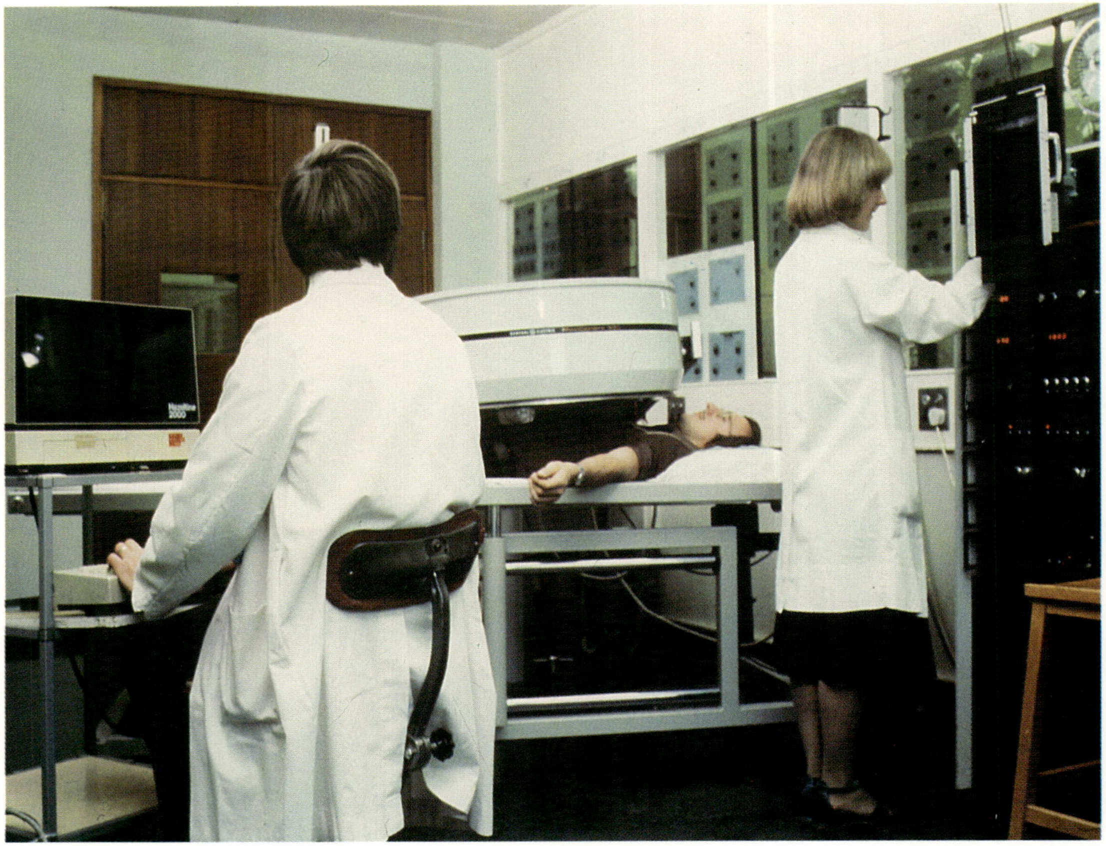

8

9

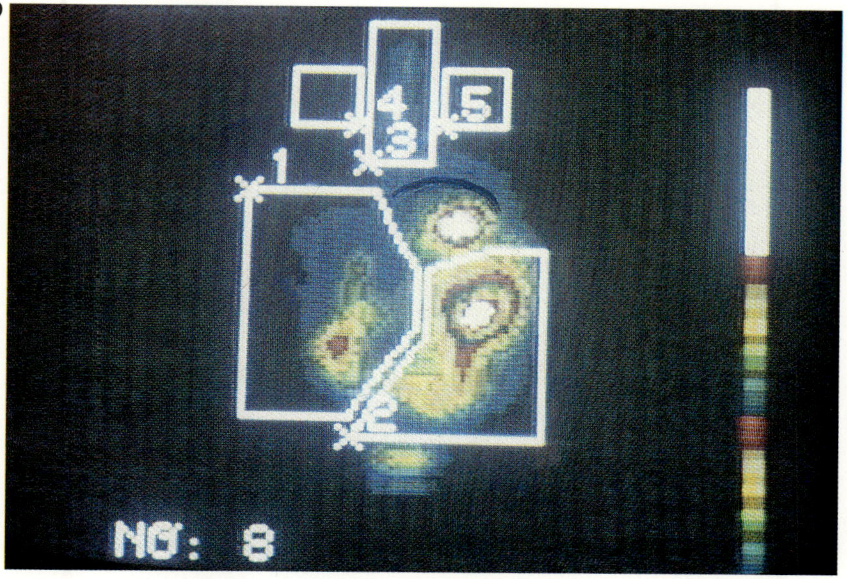

9 A computer printout of the area under the camera, 30 minutes after the injection of HIDA. In area 1 is shown the radioactivity over the liver and gall bladder. Area 2 is the majority of the radioactivity which is now in the area of the small bowel. Below 2 is a small area indicating the radioisotope in the bladder. Areas 3 and 4 are over the oesophagus and 5 is the reference area for the lung. The dense radioactivity (circled) between areas 3 and 2 indicate extensive reflux of bile into the gastric remnant in a patient who had had a Billroth II gastrectomy. The computer allows us to quantitate the amount of bile reflux occurring during the course of the test.

10

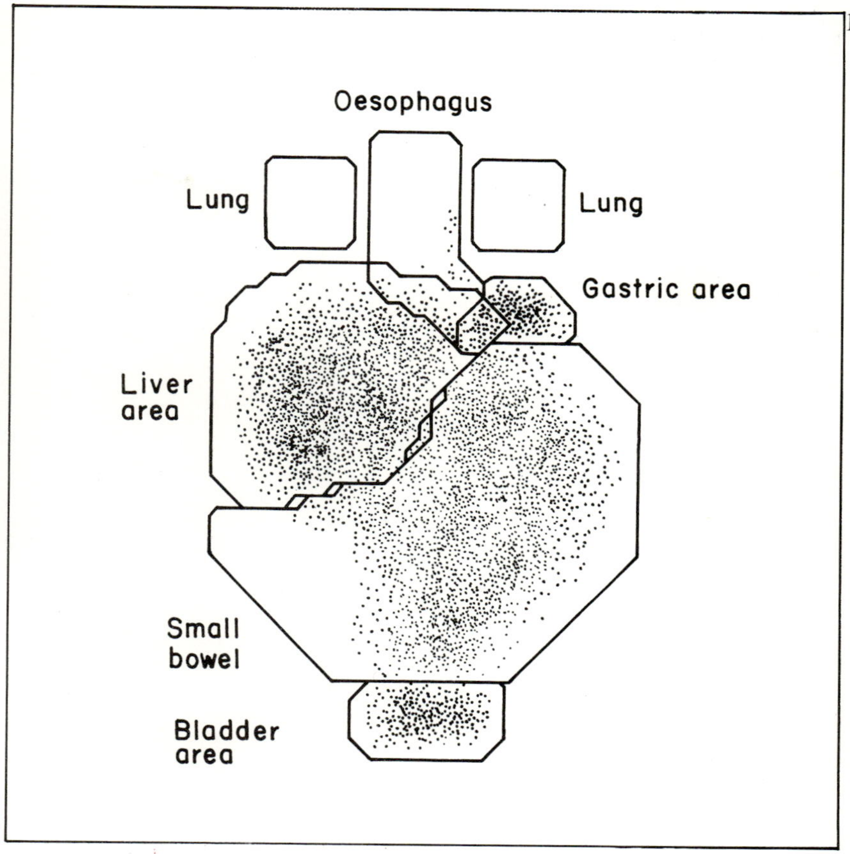

10 Printout showing isotope labelled HIDA refluxing into the gastric remnant.

NB: It is important to realise that bile reflux is intermittent and someone who may reflux no bile during the course of the 90 minute test can reflux during the night.

Preparation of patient in theatre

11 The position of the patient on the operating table, showing the pneumatic leg bags used to prevent venous stasis during the operation. These are used **instead of subcutaneous heparin which has some disadvantages,** if there is to be extensive division of adhesions within the abdomen. The operating department assistant is shown positioning the metal bridge of the automatic retractor.

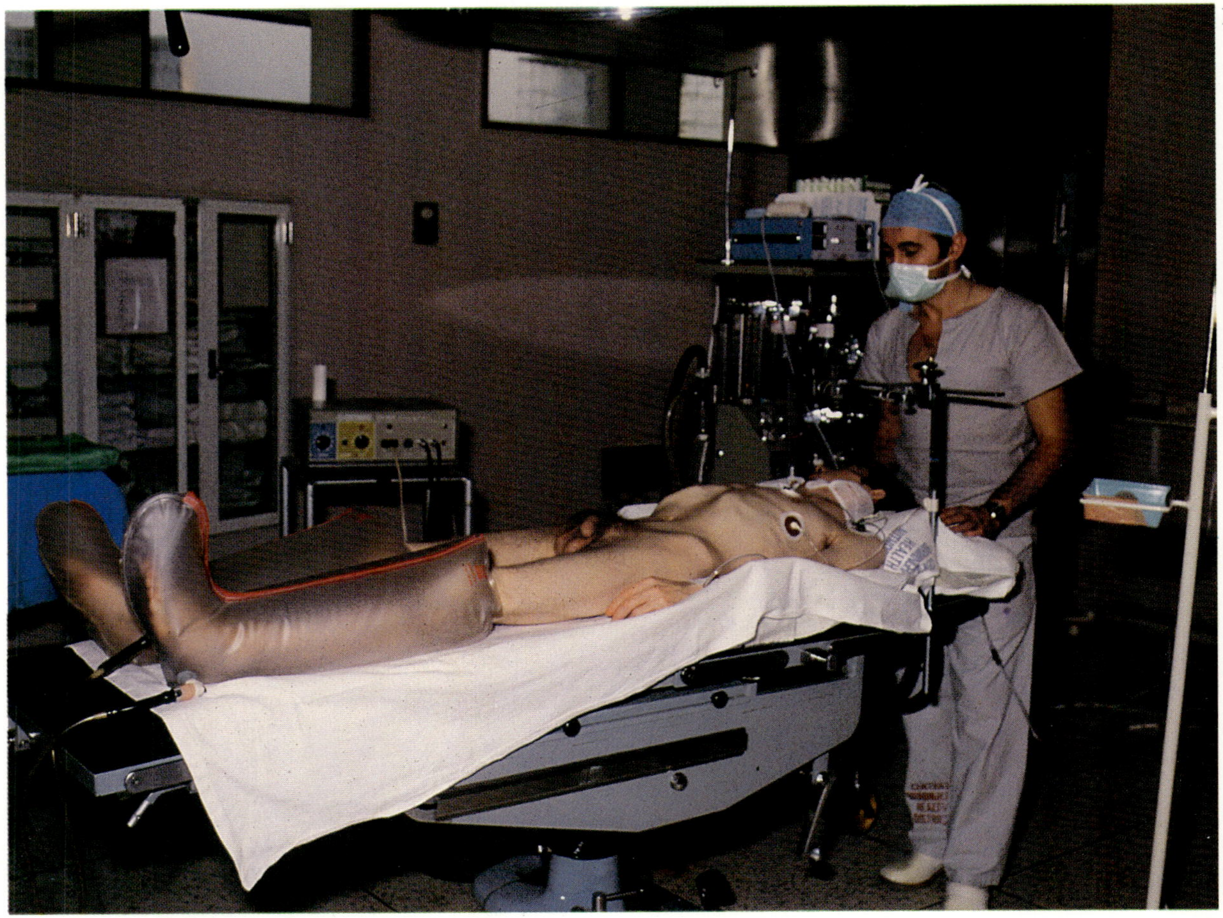

11

12

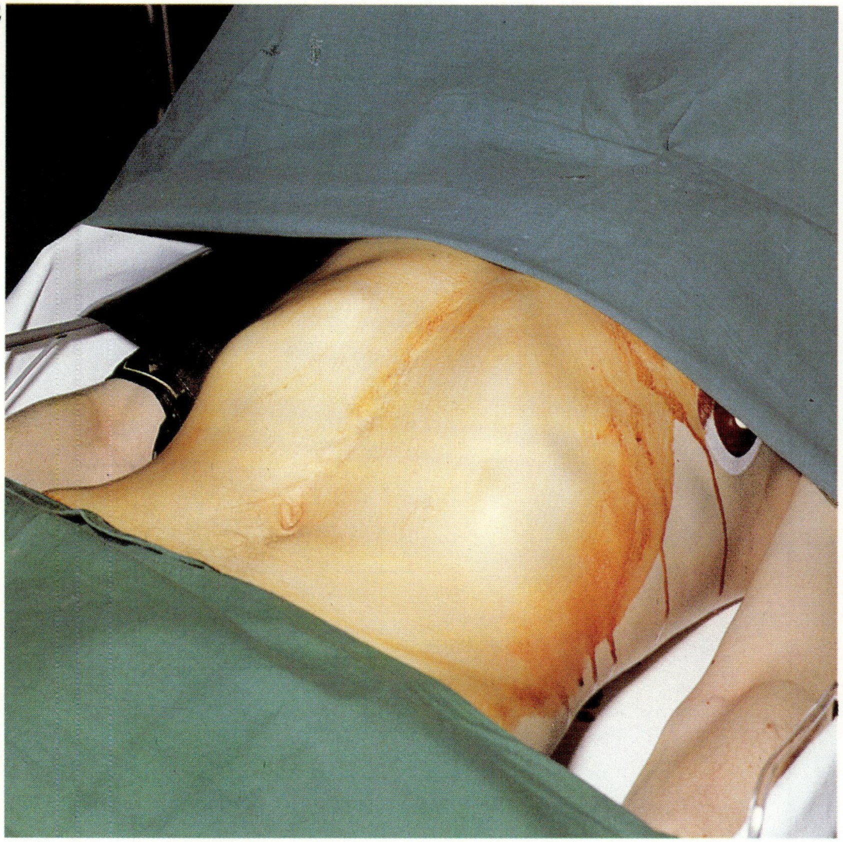

12 The patient's abdomen is shaved and prepared with an antiseptic.

13

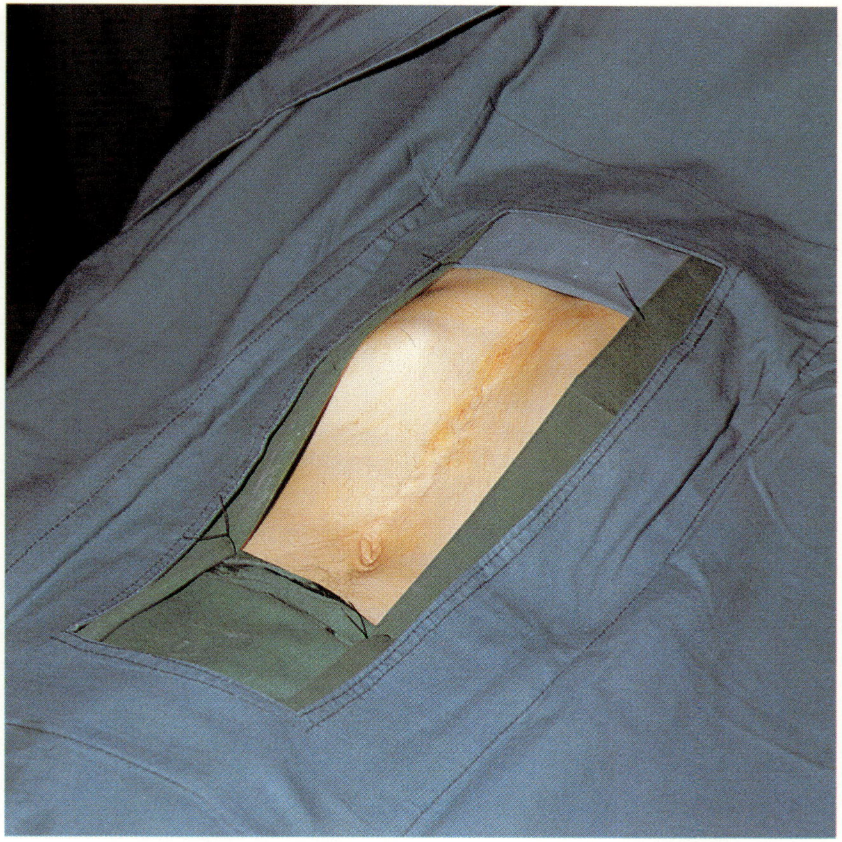

13 The relevant area of the abdomen is draped.

14 If the surgeon is righthanded, he and the nurse stand on the patient's right; the assistants are positioned on the left. Side drapes or 'wings' enable the operating team to be separated from the technical team, who will be engaged in testing the completeness of the vagotomy.

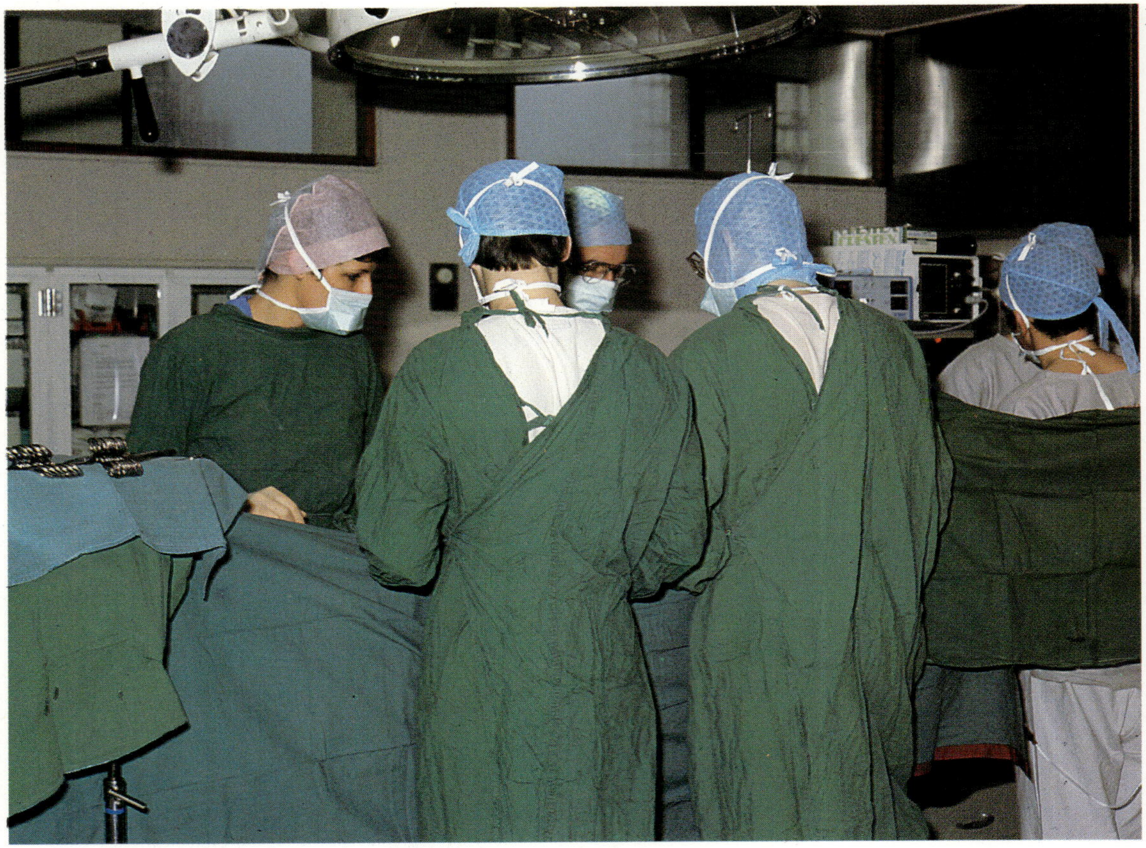

14

Entry of peritoneal cavity

15 After excising the abdominal scar and entering the peritoneal cavity, there are usually extensive adhesions to be divided. Here the linea alba is held upward with tissue forceps, putting the filmy intra-abdominal adhesions on tension so that they can be divided, usually by diathermy.

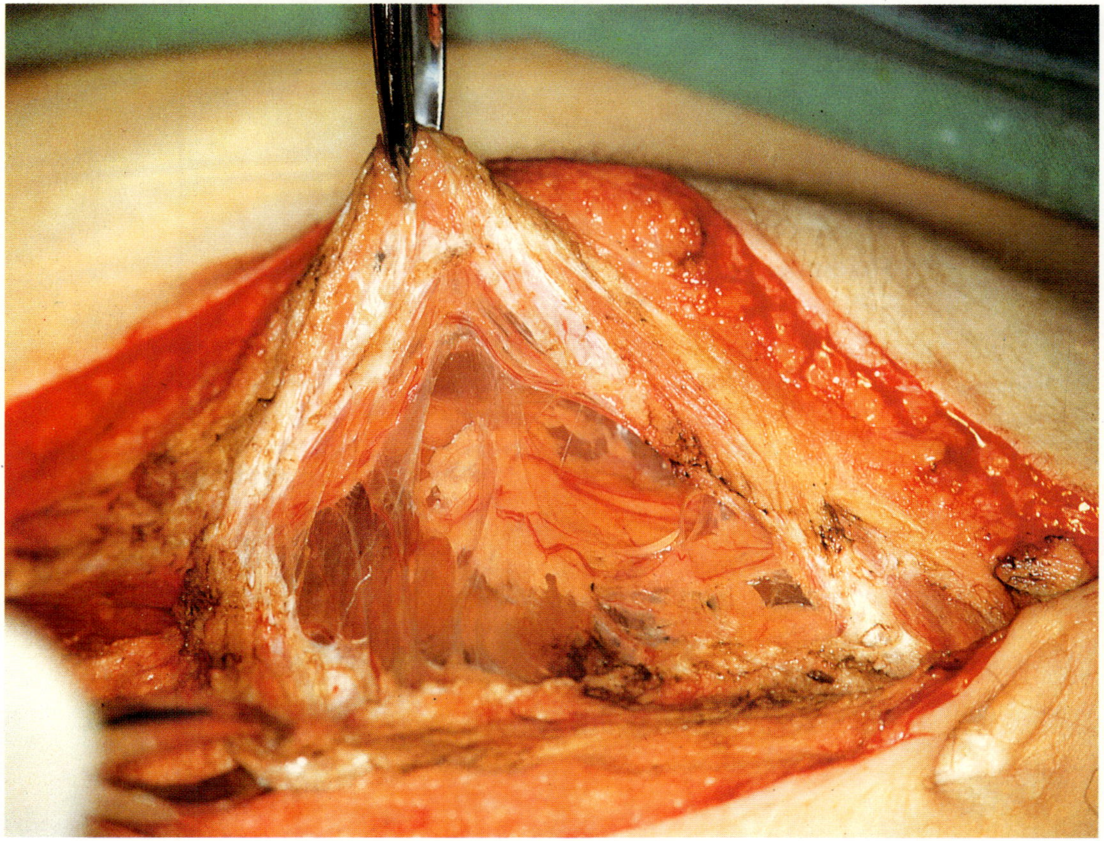

15

16 It is important to divide the coronary ligament and the filmy adhesions between the liver and diaphragm. This is particularly important if the vagotomy is to be repeated.

16

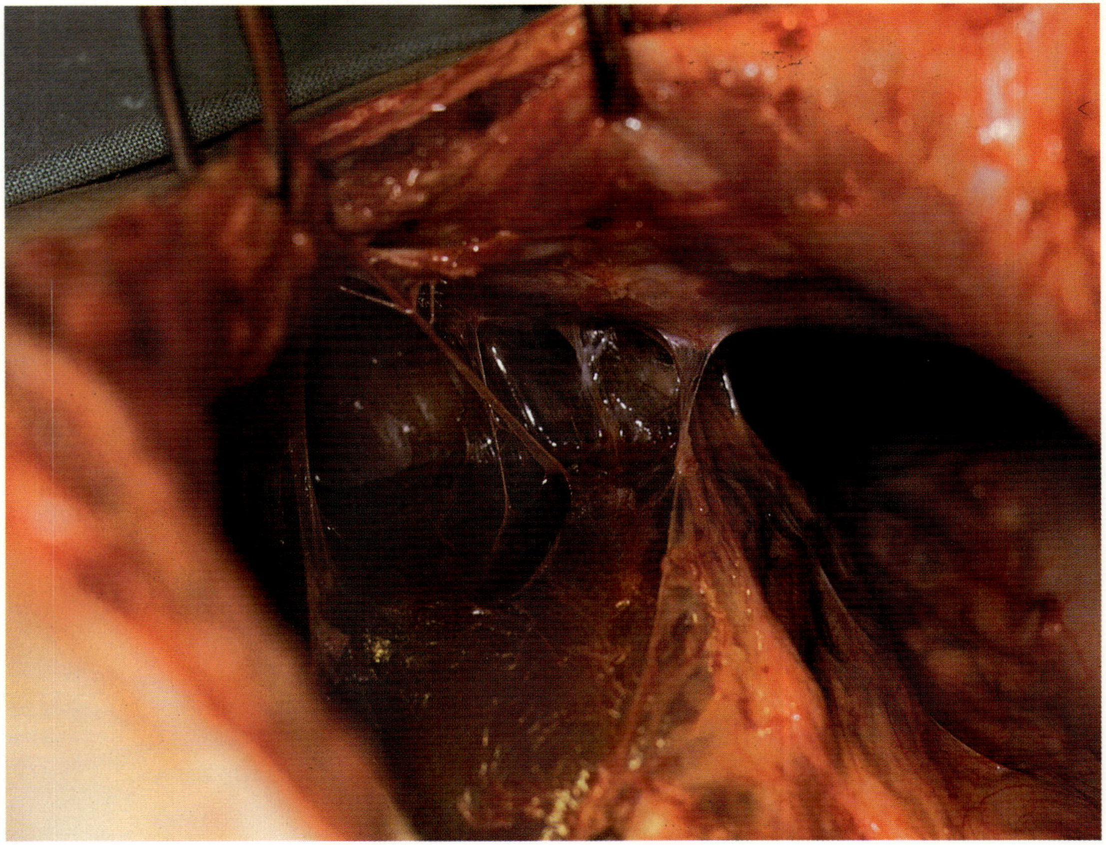

17

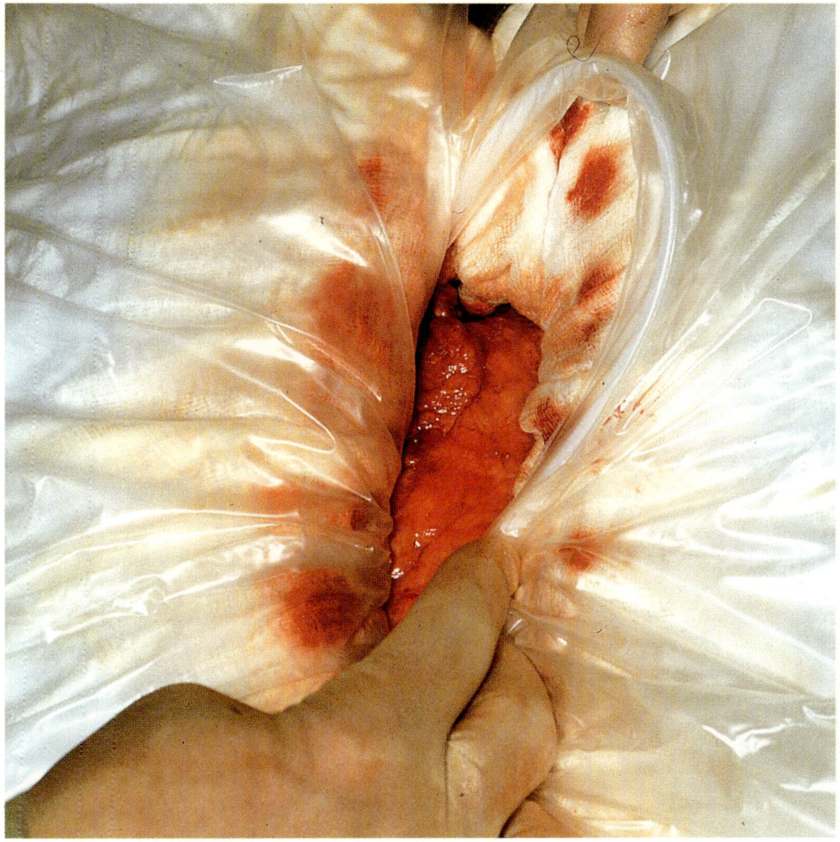

18

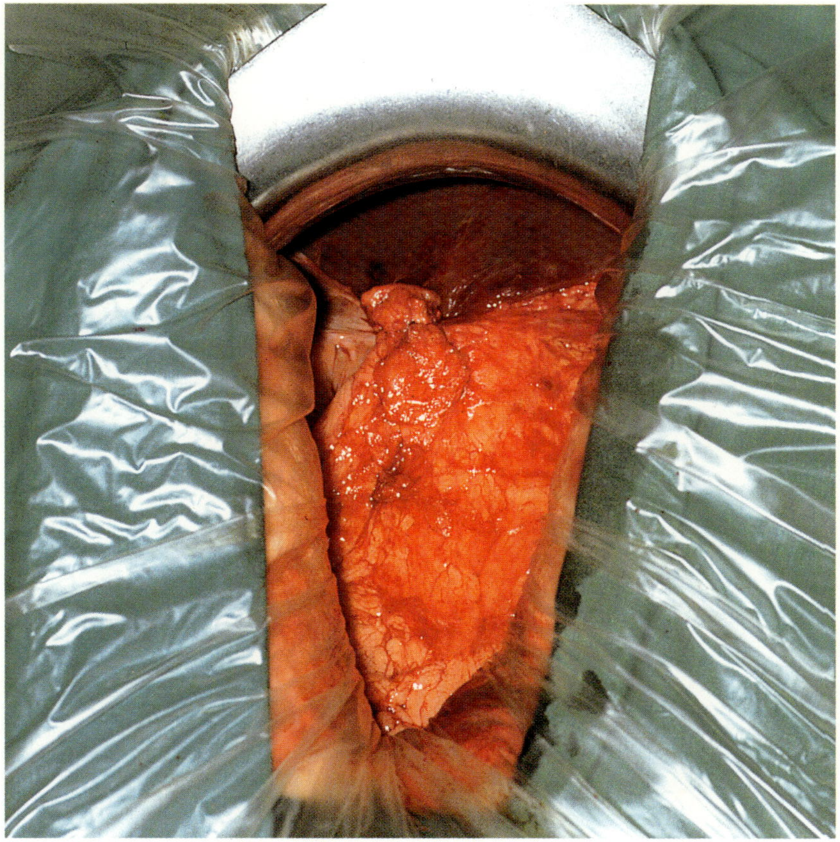

17 Once all the intra-abdominal adhesions have been freed, antiseptic impregnated wound-guards are used to protect the wound edge and a 7 or 9 inch plastic wound drape is inserted.

18 The medium-sized blade of the Rochard automatic retractor is used to pull up the upper part of the wound and the costal margin.

19 The retractor is attached to the metal bridge to give vertical and cranial traction. The lower part of the wound is spread with another self-retaining retractor.

19

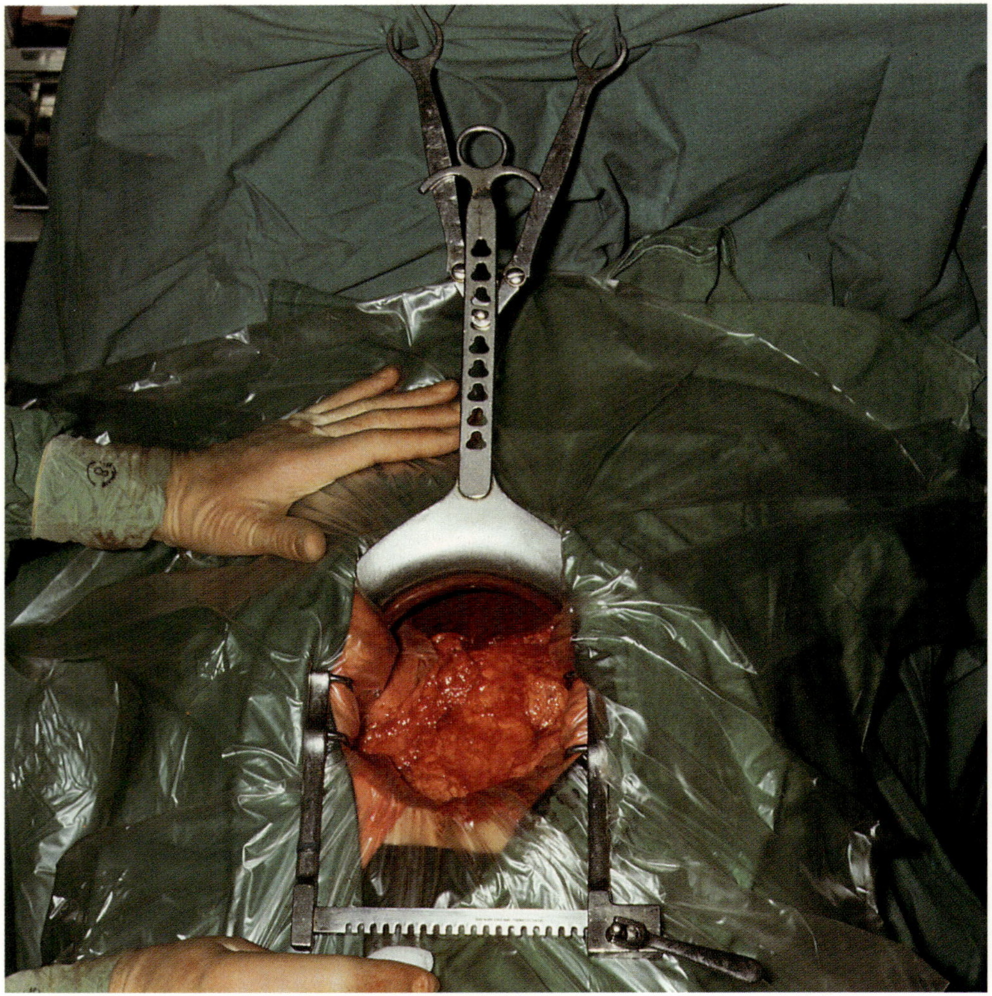

20

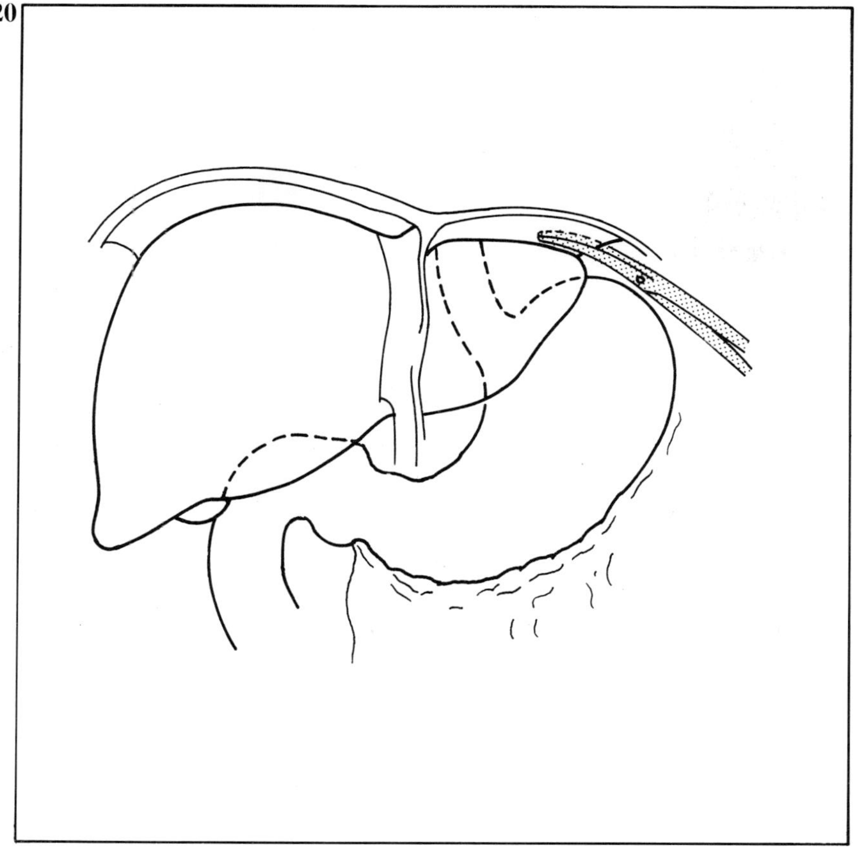

20 Diagram showing the division of the left coronary ligament of the liver.

21

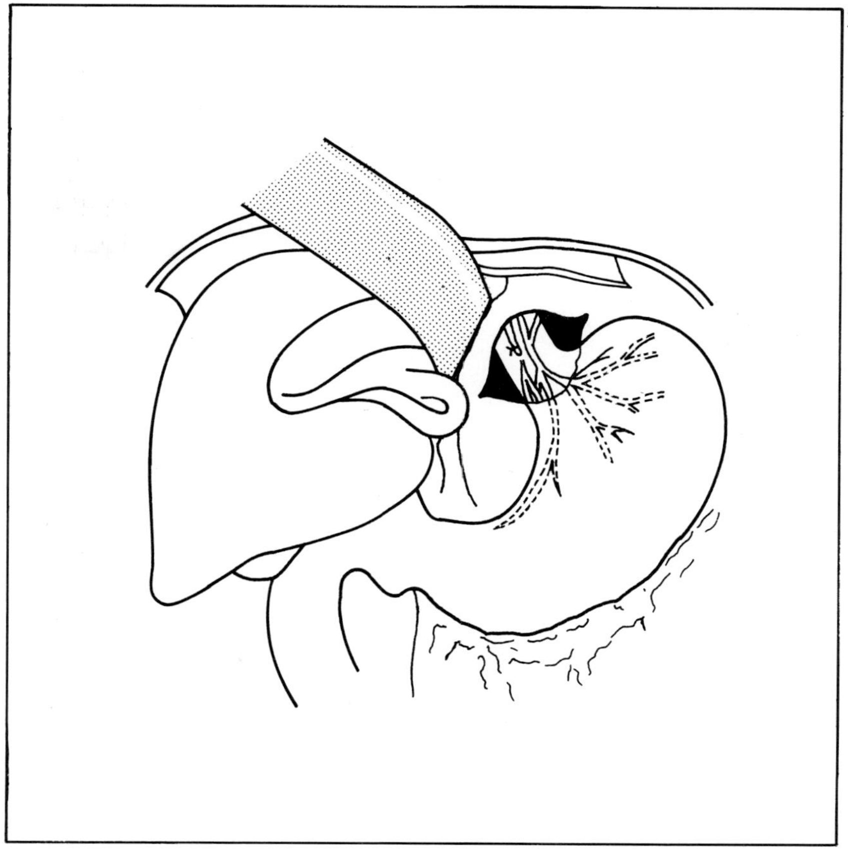

21 After dividing the coronary ligament, the left lobe of the liver is rotated to the right to allow the peritoneum over the oesophagogastric junction to be divided.

Performing and testing the vagotomy

22 After dividing the left coronary ligament of the liver and displacing the left lobe of the liver towards the right, the oesophagus is dissected with precision. **The oesophagus can often best be located and isolated by touch,** sometimes aided by the presence of a tube in the oesophagus. Once the oesophagus is identified, it is mobilised and lifted forward by the index finger of the left hand (of a righthanded surgeon).

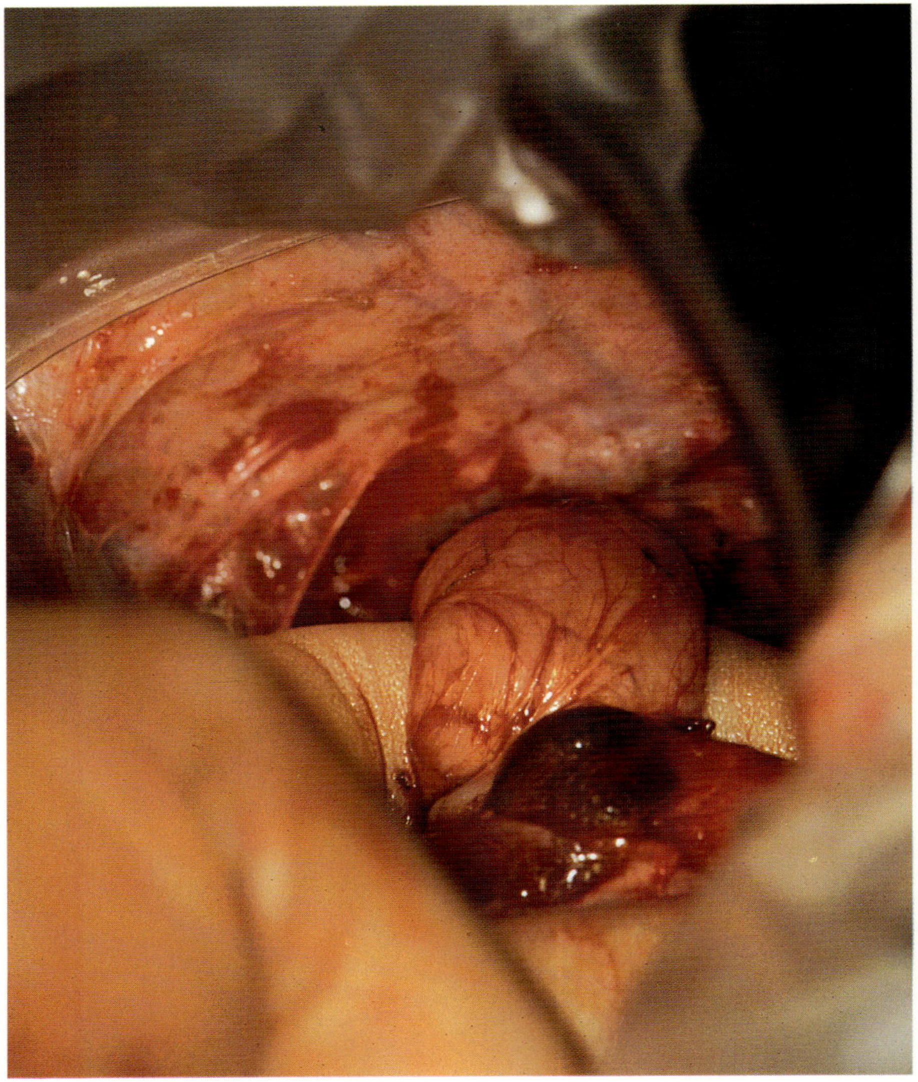
22

23

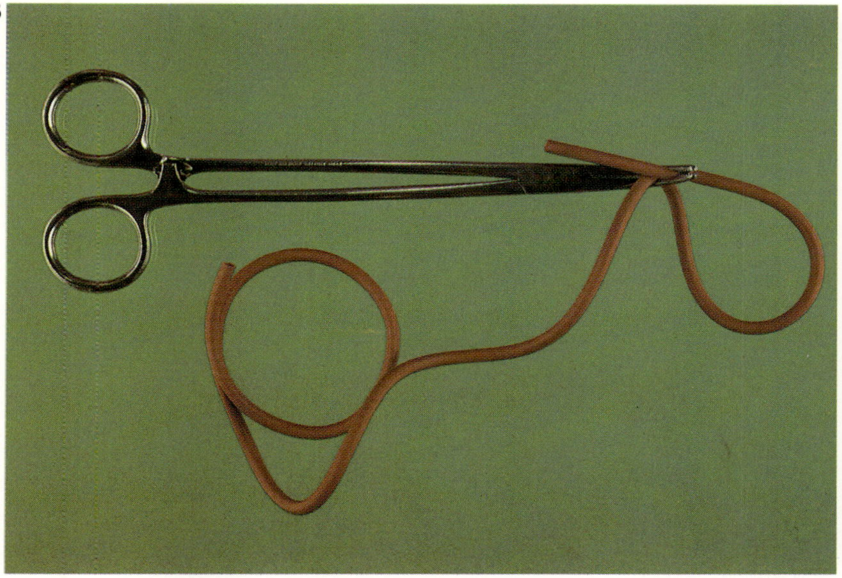

23 A length of thin rubber tubing has a small loop created near its one end.

24

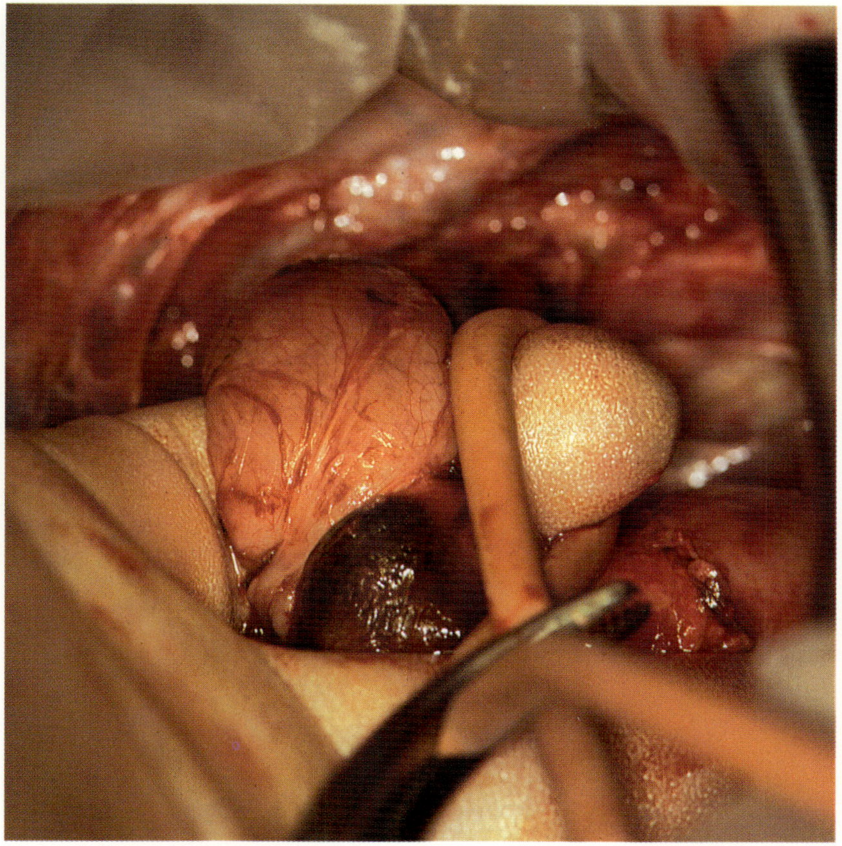

24 The loop is passed down to the right of the oesophagus and engages round the tip of the index finger that encircles the oesophagus.

25 **The finger-tip is flipped backwards to the left bringing the loop of tubing with it.**

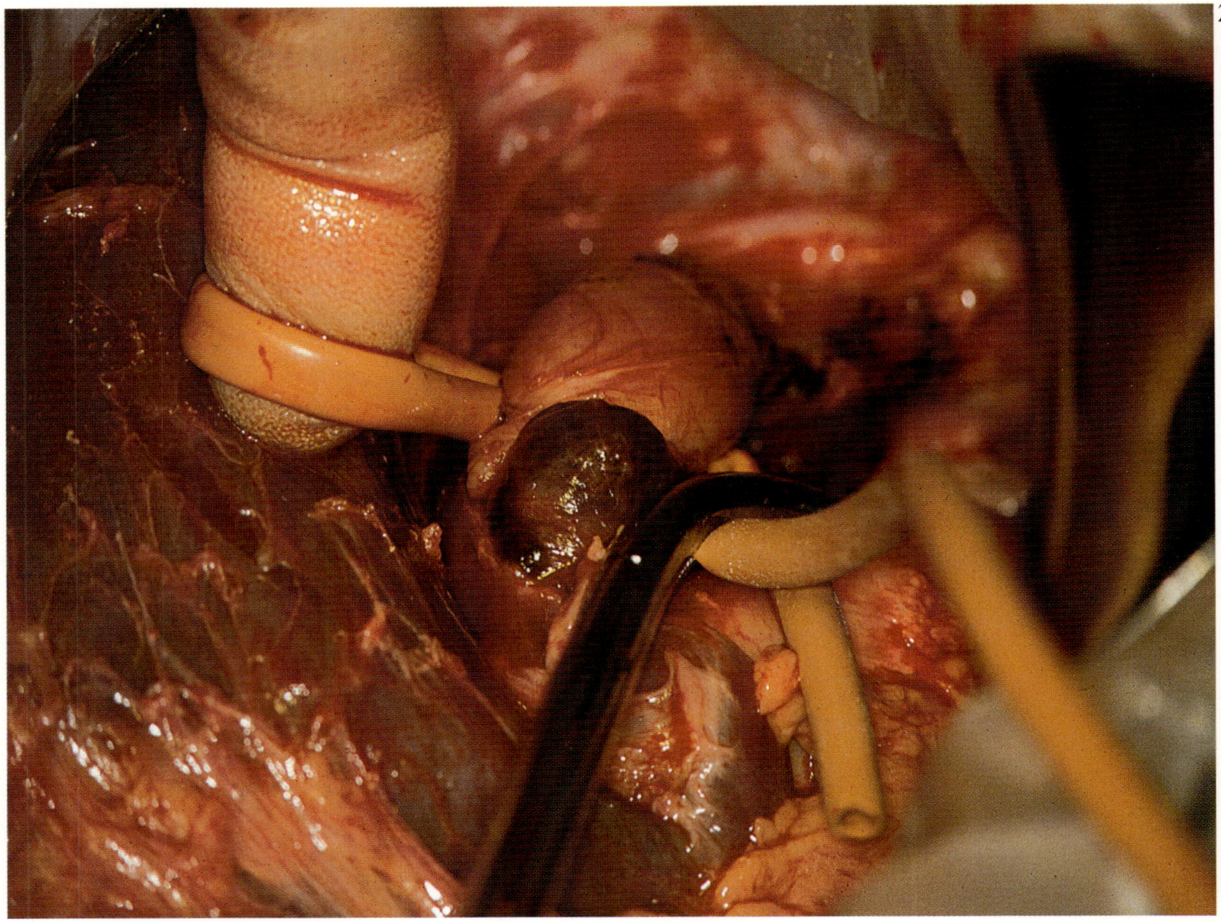

25

26 The rubber tubing encircles the oesophagus and any residual vagal fibres, holding them forward.

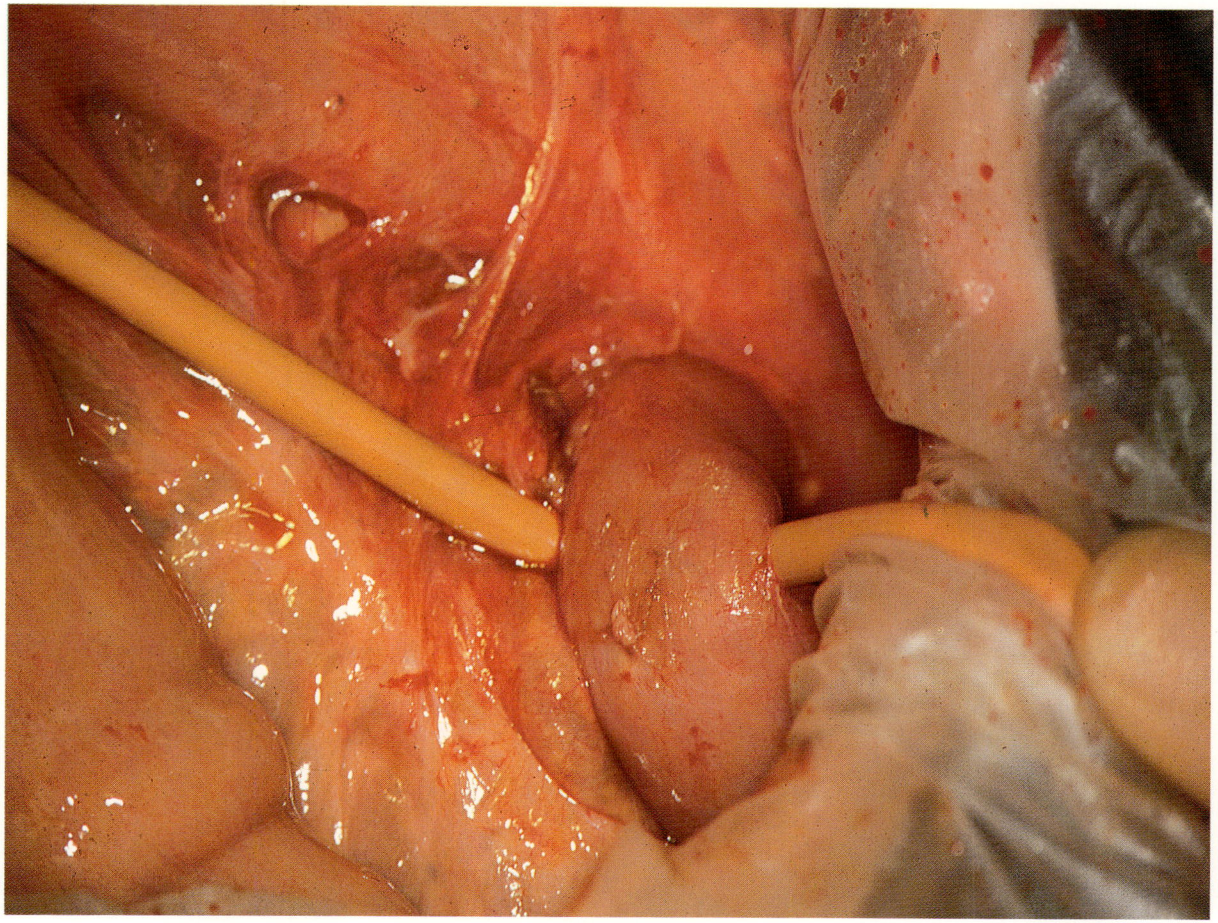
26

27

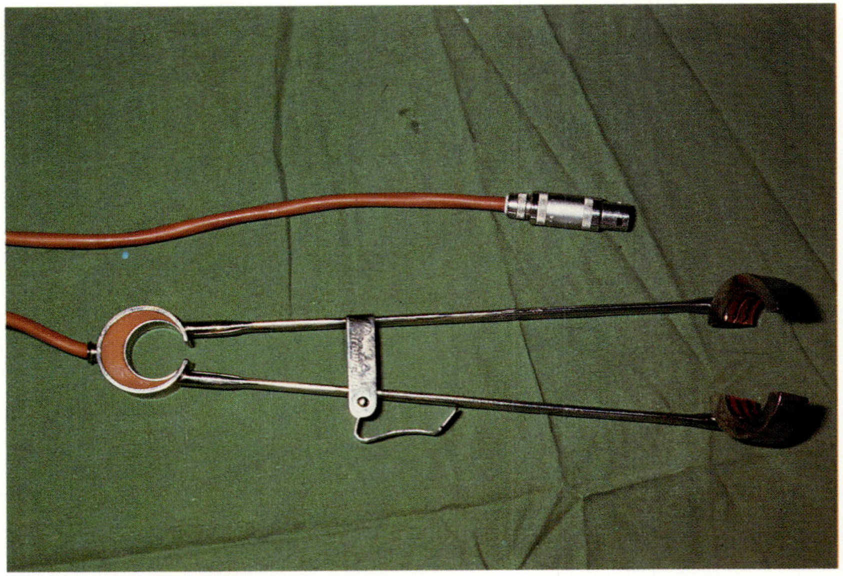

28

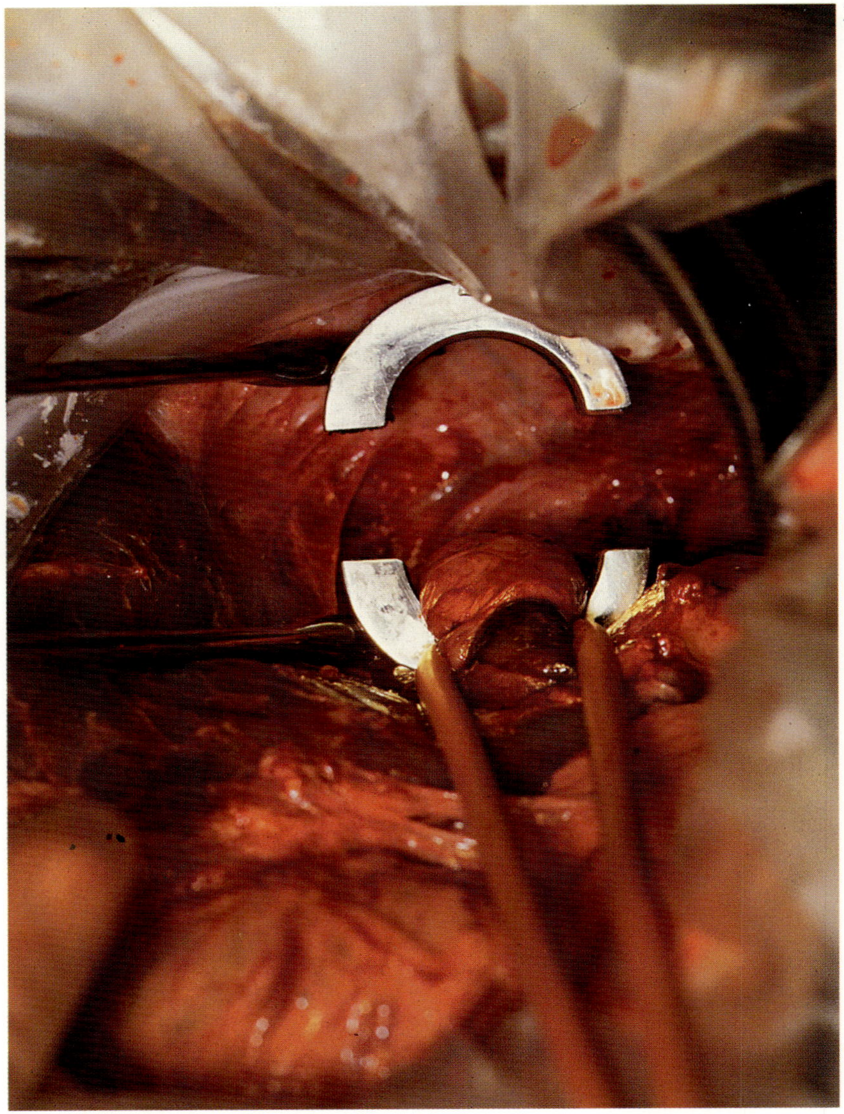

27 The encircling electrode or 'calipers' of the Vagorec testing machine have been prepared by ethyleneoxide or liquid antiseptic sterilization. Two encircling electrode rings, 1 cm apart, are located in the distal end of the calipers.

28 Using the rubber sling to hold the oesophagus upwards, the posterior part of the caliper is placed around the oesophagus.

29

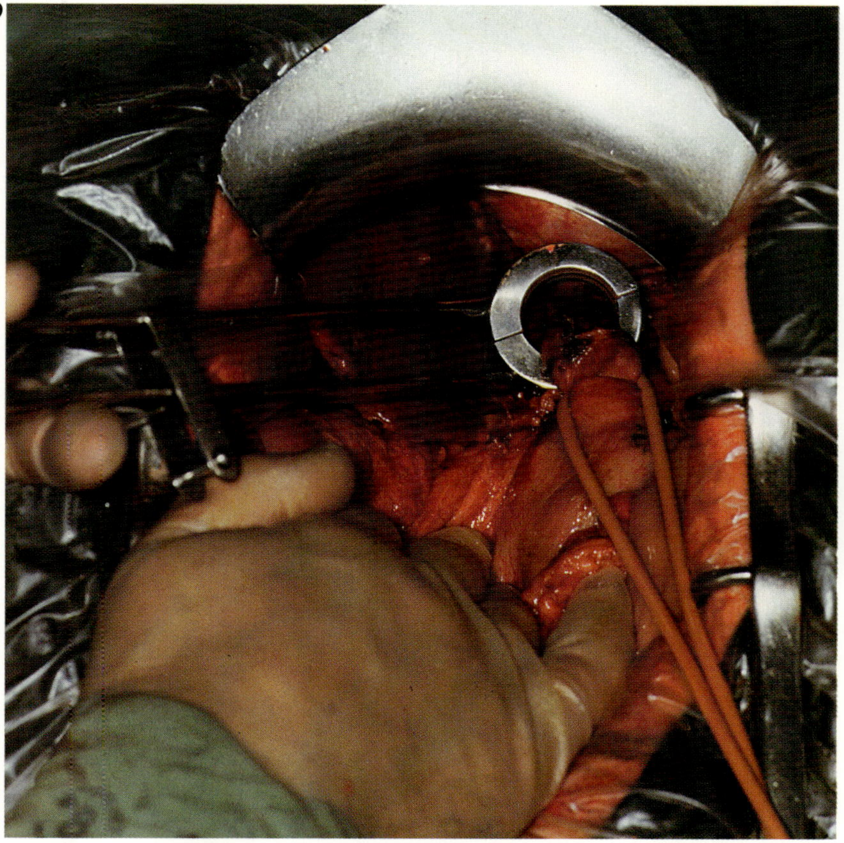

30

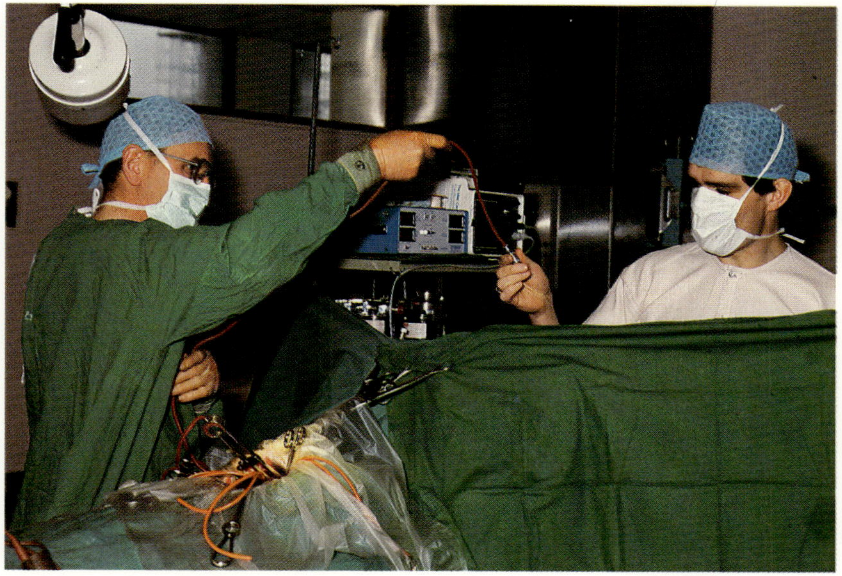

30 The end of the electrical lead is then passed to the assistant to be connected to the Vagorec machine.

29 The calipers are closed to give complete encirclement of the oesophagus. The large bore oesophageal tube is then passed down the oesophagus through the electrode. The balloon of the tube, when inflated, will compress the edge of the oesophagus and the vagi against the metal part of the electrode.

31

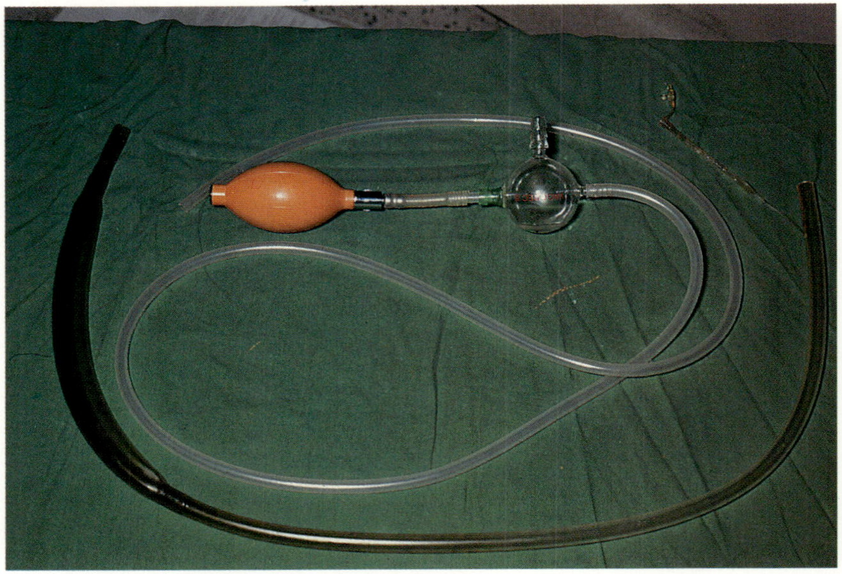

32

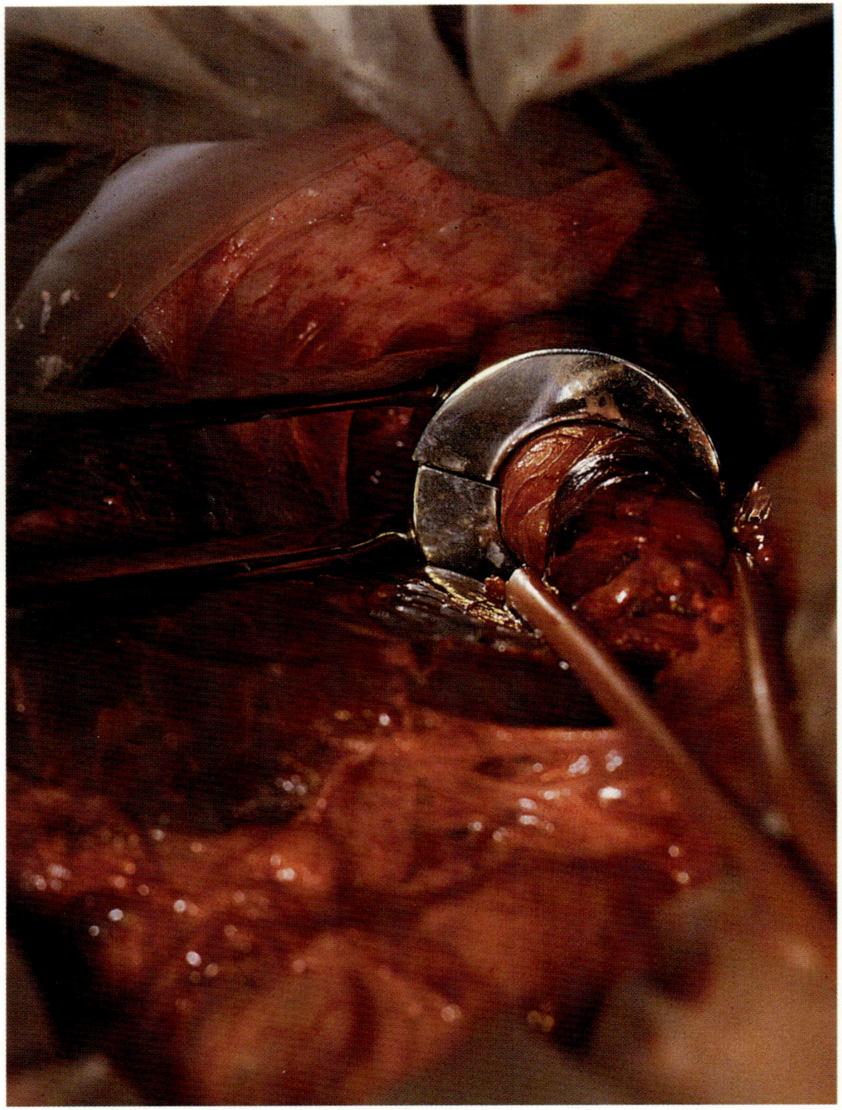

31 The assistant then assembles the gastro-oesophageal tube with its associated gastric inflation bulb, saliva trap and balloon-inflation tube.

32 This tube is then passed down the oesophagus through the electrode until it extends for about 10 cm into the stomach or gastric remnant.

33 Diagram of the assembly of the Vagorec apparatus showing the wide-bore tube, with its inflatable cuff, placed in the stomach with the lower oesophagus surrounded by the electrodes. A soft clamp is placed across the junction between the antrum and the body of the stomach and another clamp across the duodenum distal to the pylorus.

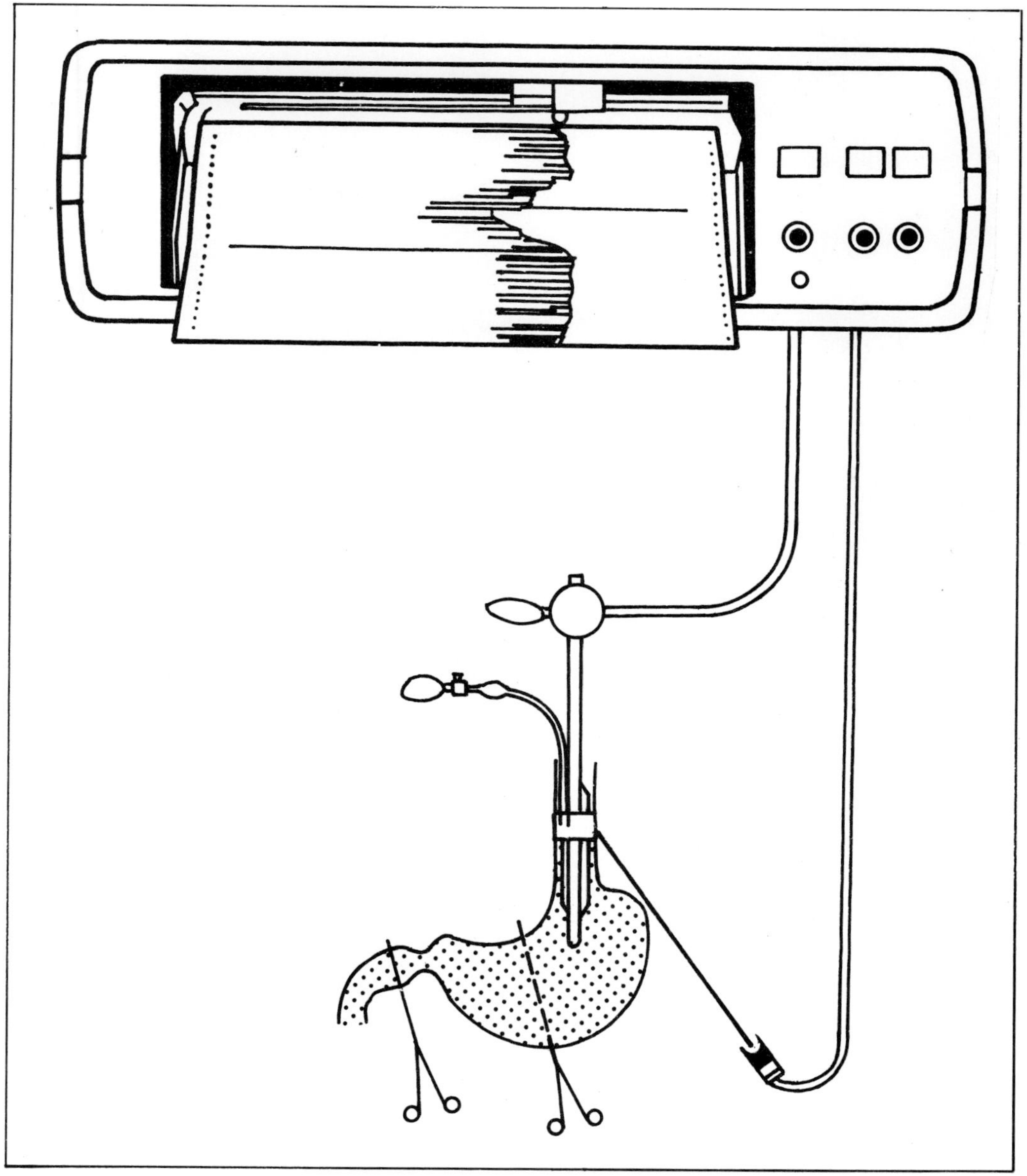

33

34

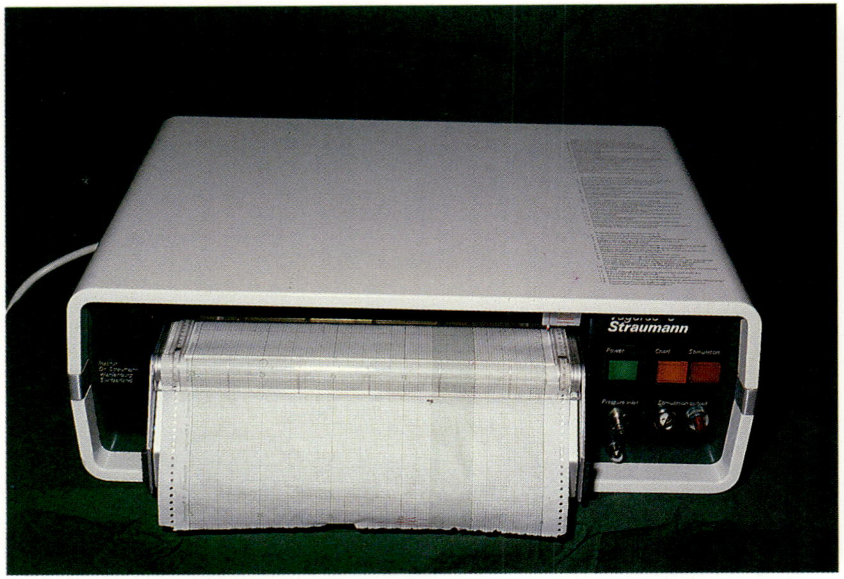

34 The pen tracing machine that registers the intragastric pressure.

35

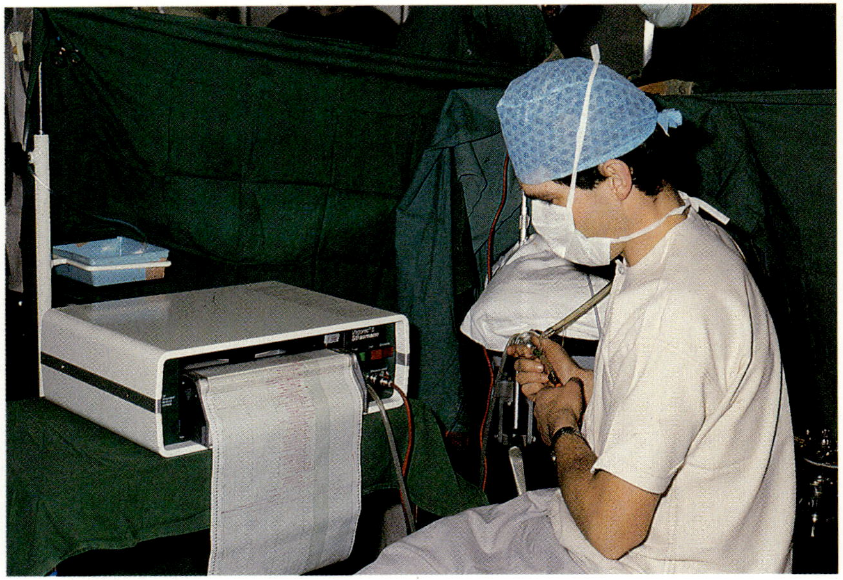

35 The assistant inflating the stomach with air until the pressure recorded fits in, or near, the green band on the tracing paper.

36

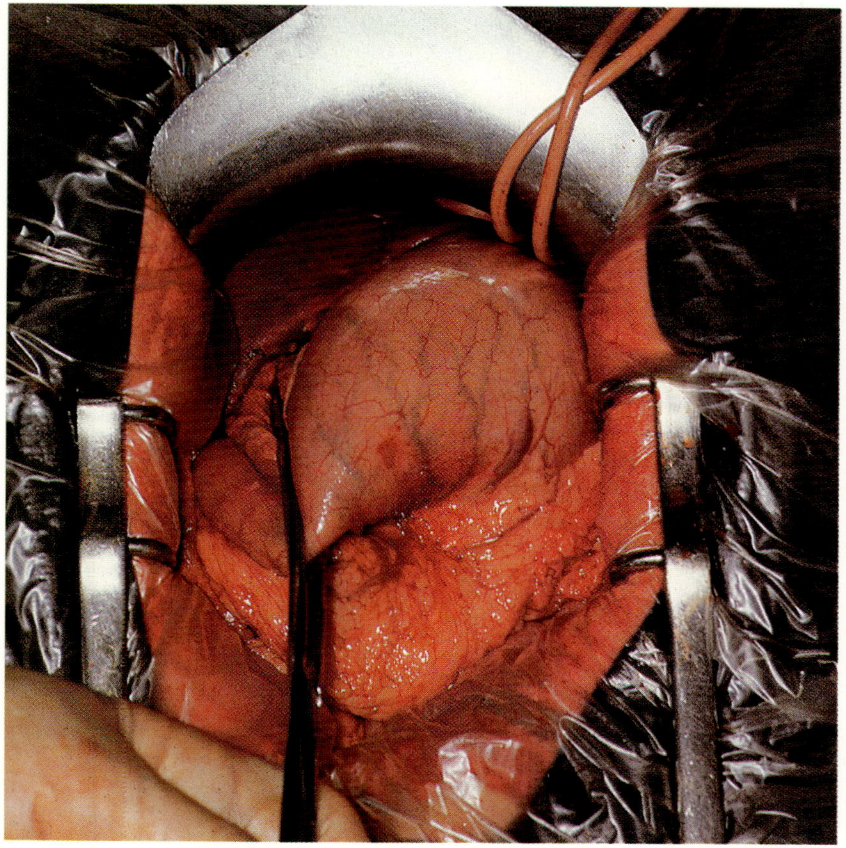

36 The stomach inflated with air proximal to the soft clamp placed between the antrum and body of the stomach.

37

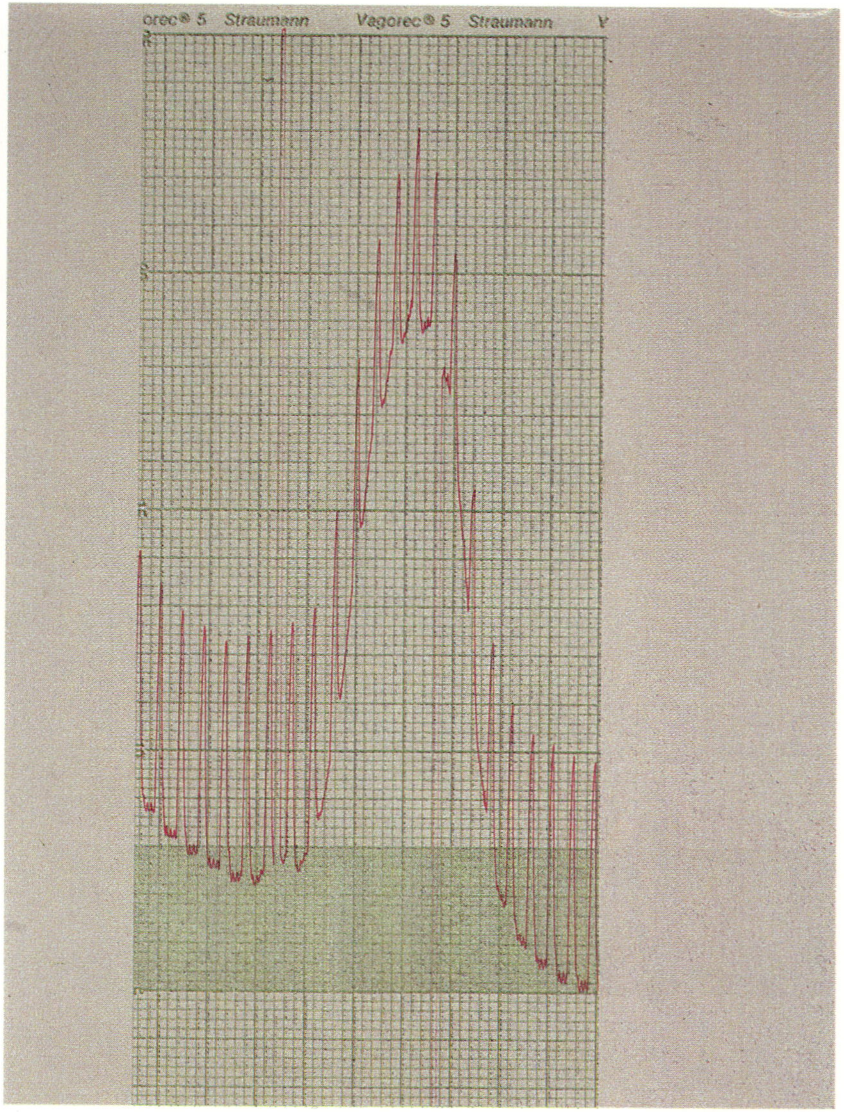

37 A typical tracing of the pressure rise in the stomach following electrical stimulation of intact vagi.

38

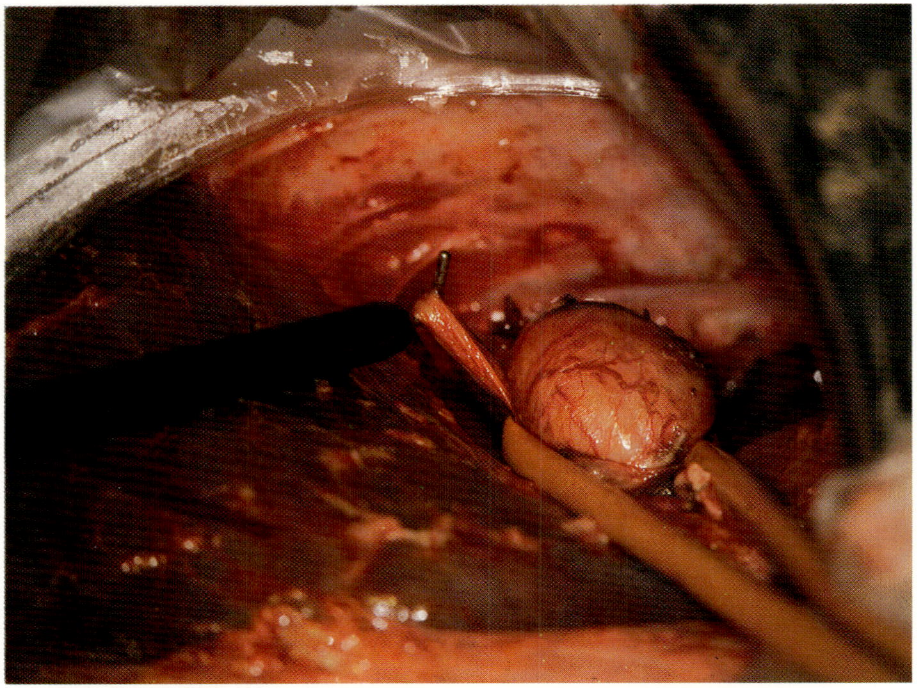

39

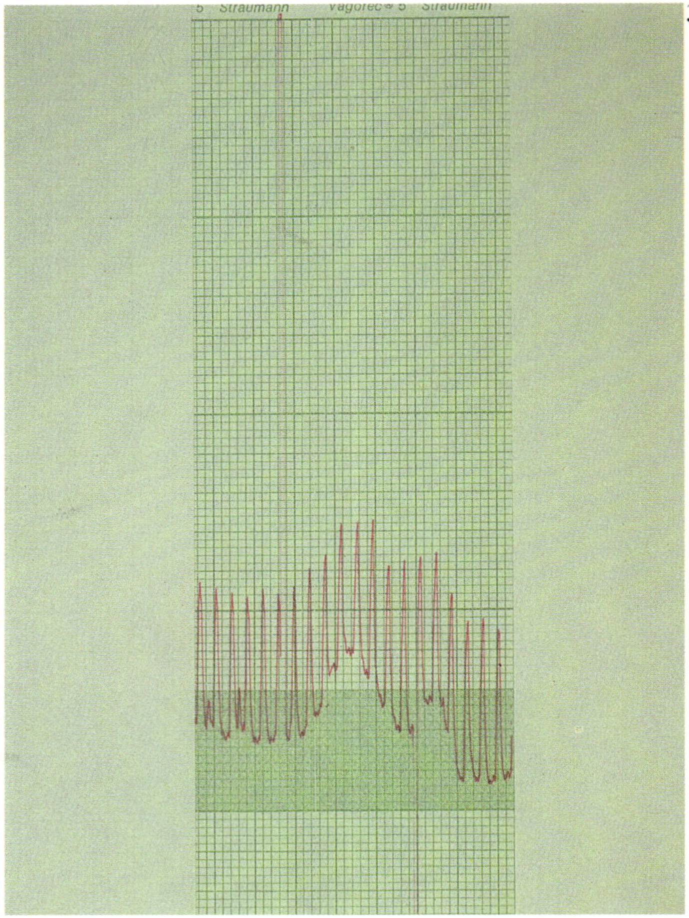

38 In this patient the large posterior vagal trunk is located with an insulated vagotomy nerve hook. This hook is used for diathermy destruction (see below).

39 After division of the posterior vagus the gastric pressure response is almost abolished but a small response is still evident. Therefore, a search for further nerve fibres is undertaken.

40 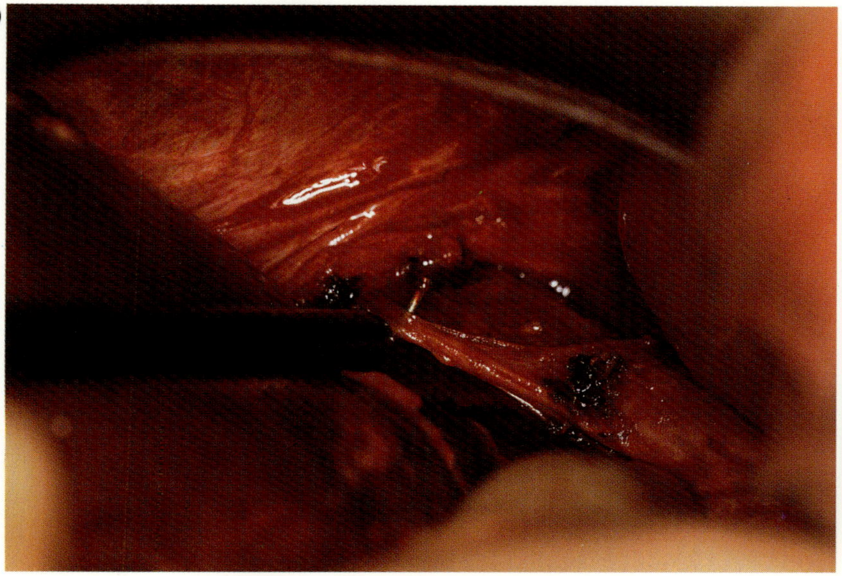

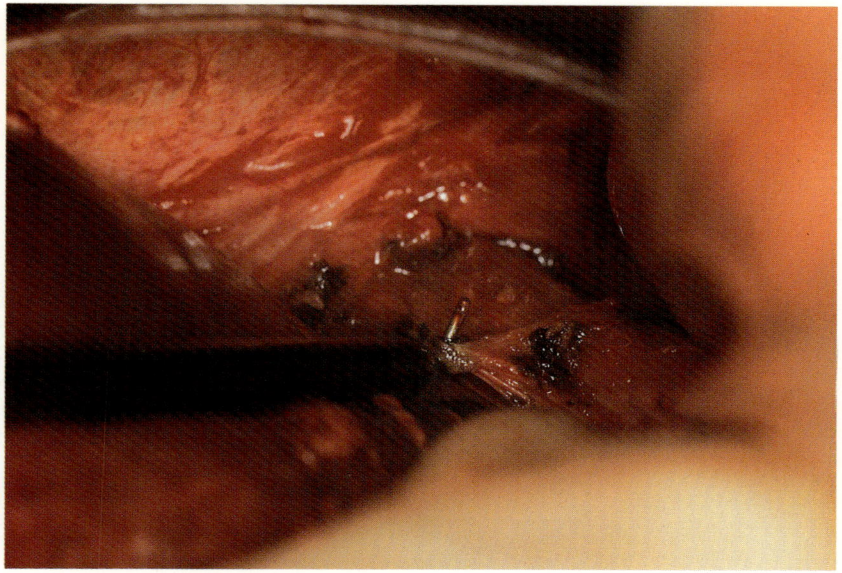 41

40 A small anterior vagal nerve fibre is located and lifted up with the nerve hook.

41 The nerve is destroyed by electrical diathermy coagulation distally.

42 The nerve hook is then slid up the nerve proximally and a second coagulation current is passed. The charred area of the nerve in the centre is divided.

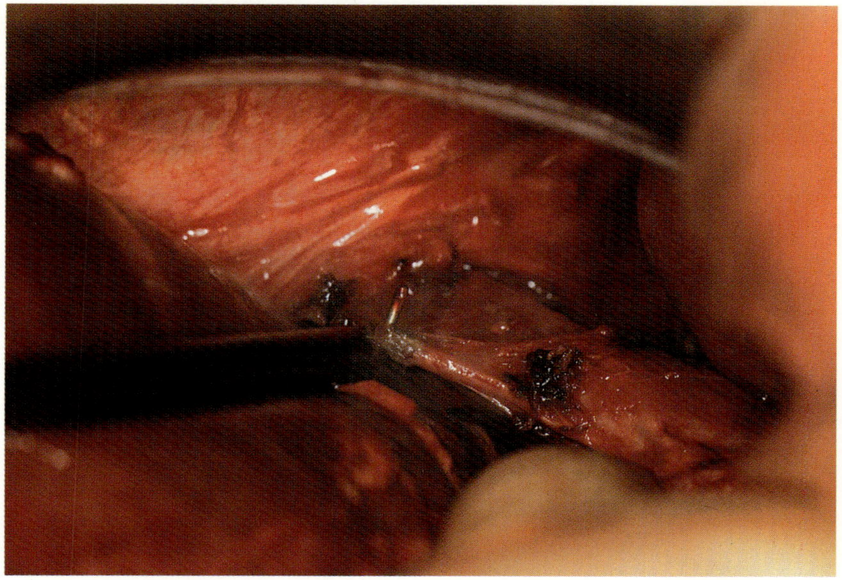 42

43

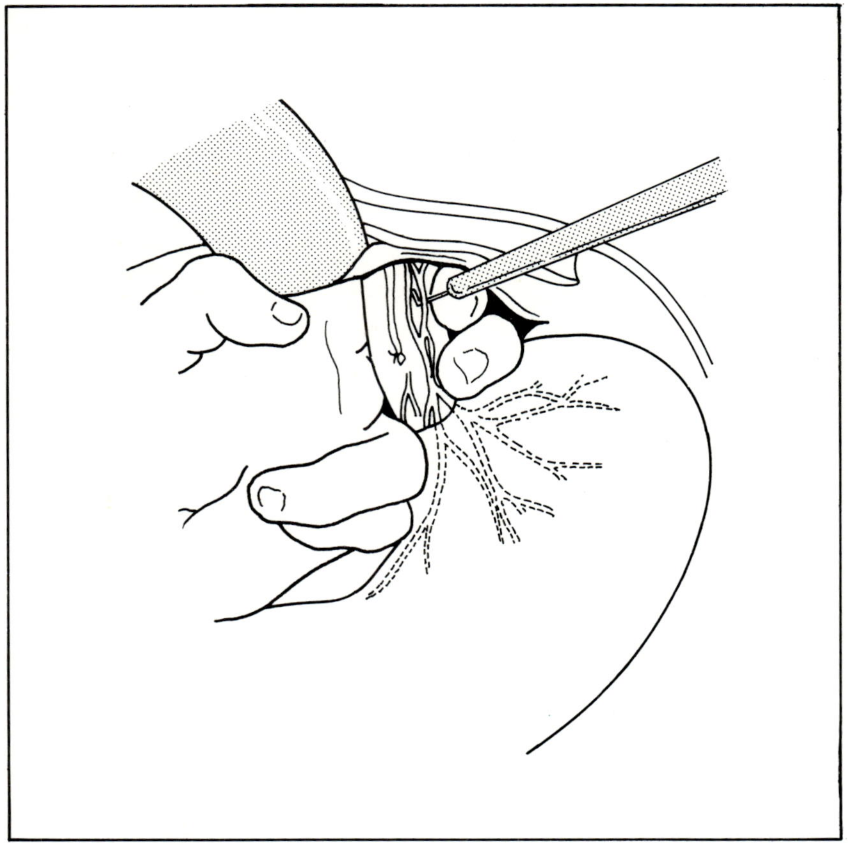

43 **Diathermy of other small residual vagal fibres.**

44

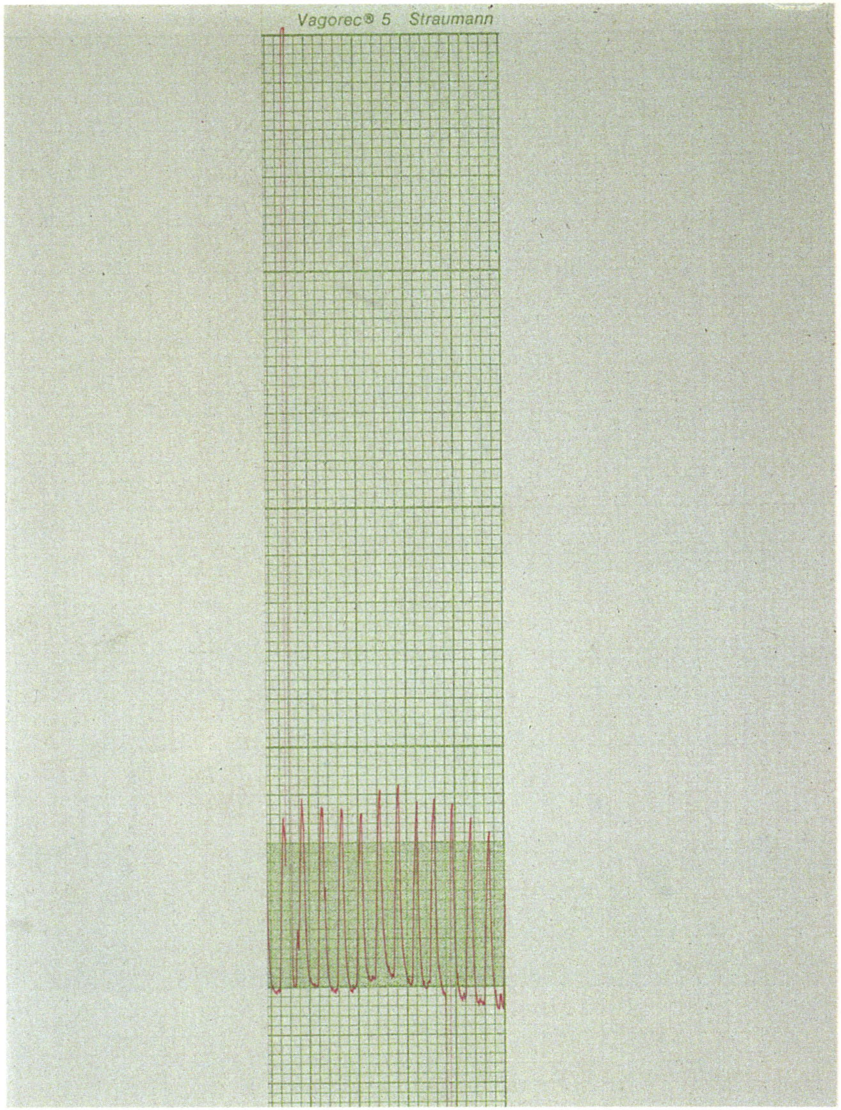

44 This manoeuvre has now completely abolished the motor response of the stomach to electrical stimulation indicating the complete vagotomy.

45 **The abdominal oesophagus with all the small vagal fibres divided is now free and mobile.**

45

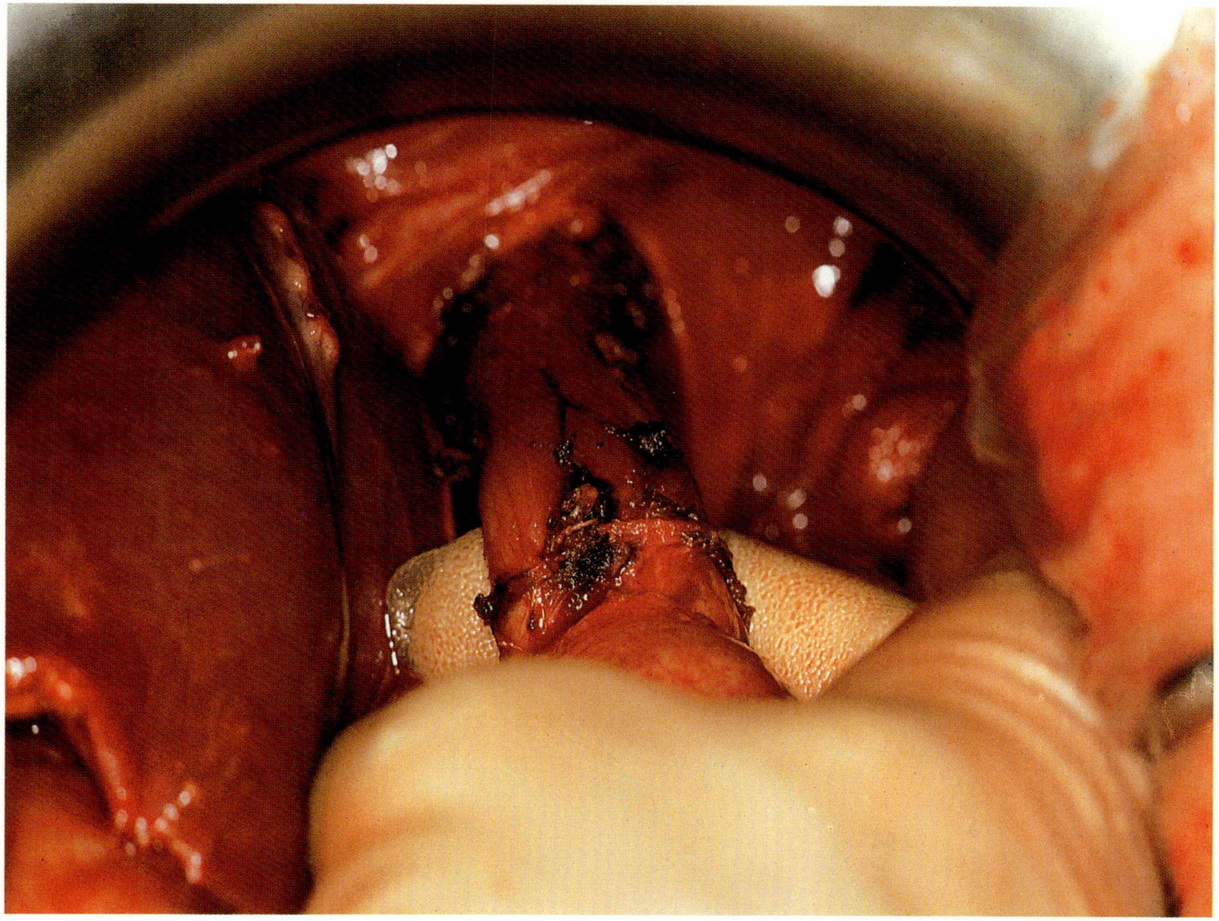

Division of duodenum before antrectomy

46

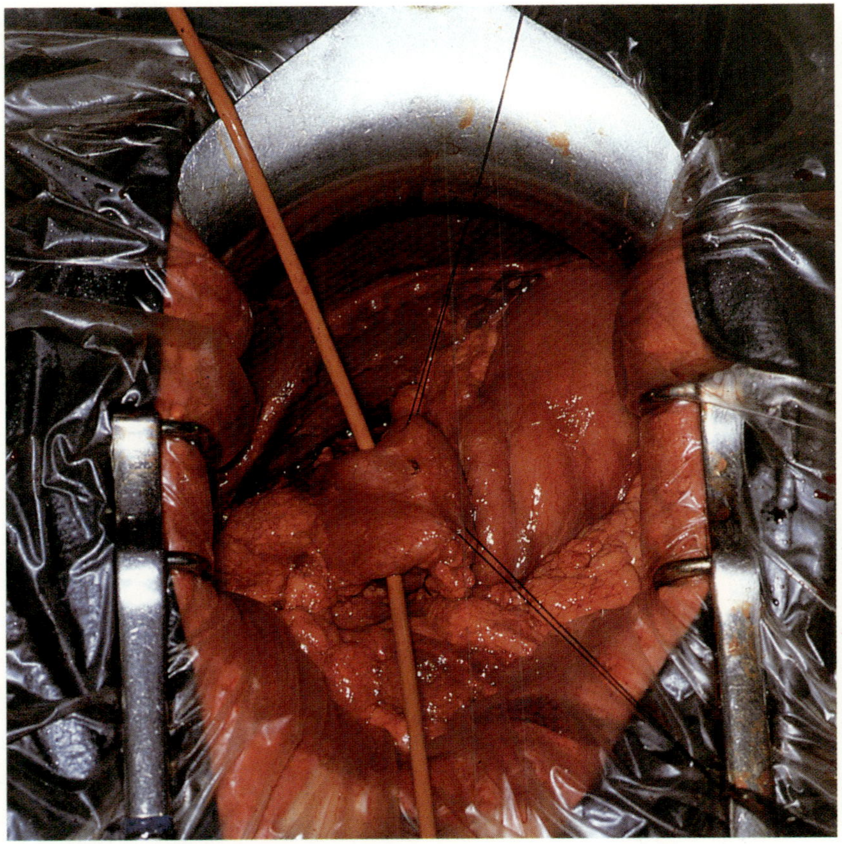

46 This patient had a previous vagotomy and pyloroplasty and is about to have the duodenum divided to perform an antrectomy. Division of the duodenum is facilitated if another tube can be passed behind the duodenum just beyond the pyloroplasty. The site of the previous pyloroplasty is held up by stay-sutures.

47

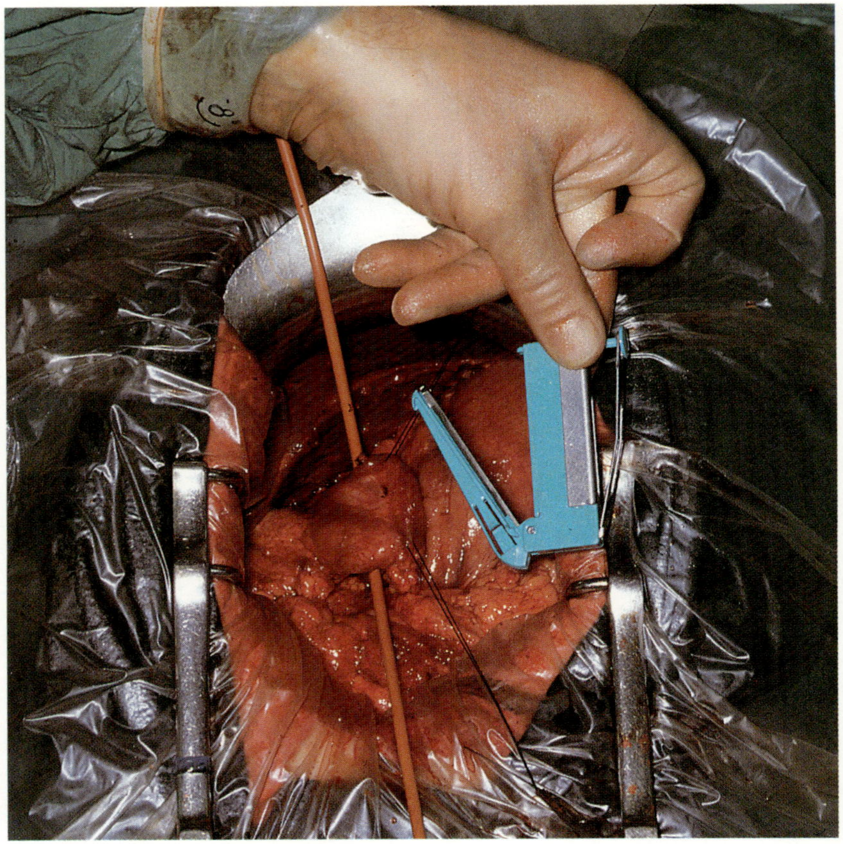

47 Traction on the rubber tube enables the duodenum to be pulled forward so that a stapling device can be placed behind it.

48

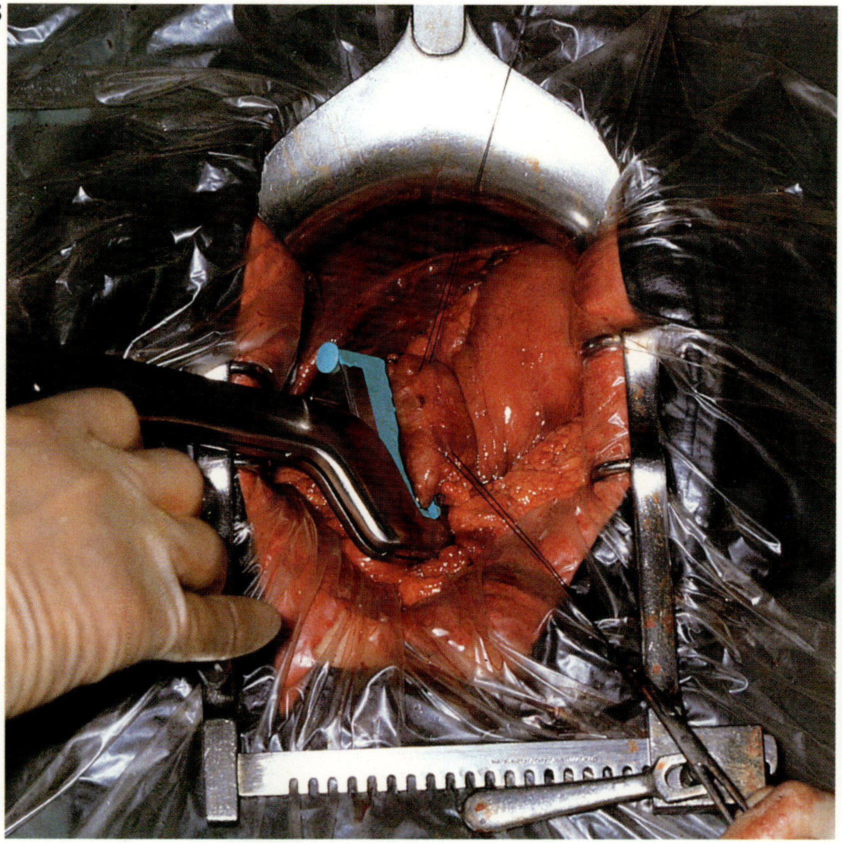

48 The TA 55 stapling gun occludes the first part of the duodenum with two layers of staples.

49

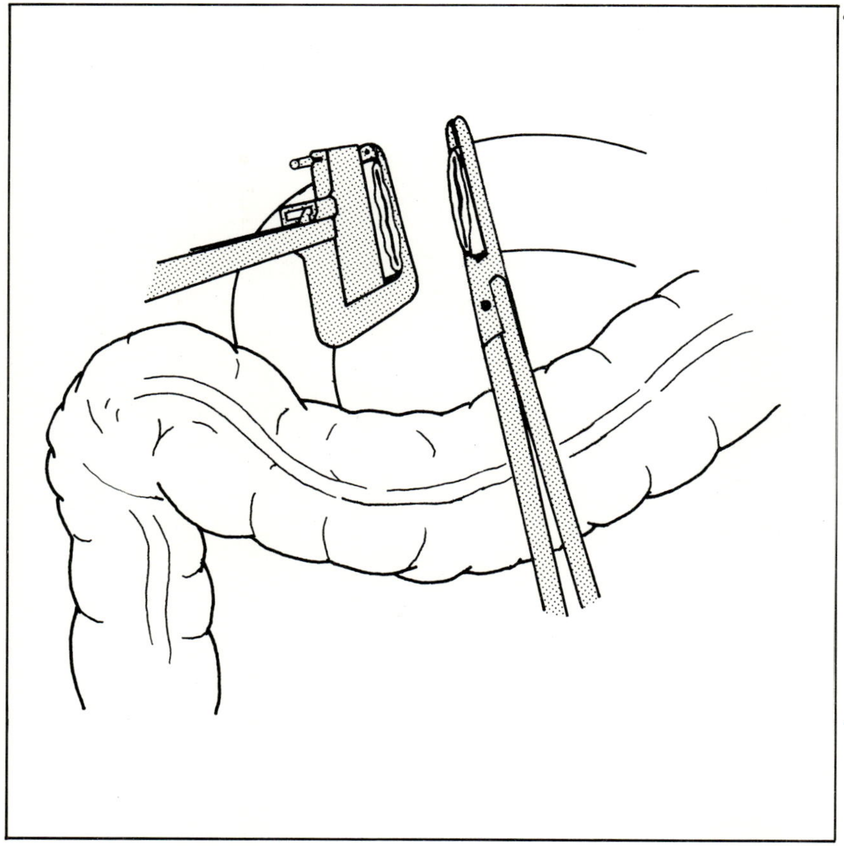

49 The duodenal stump is closed with a TA 55 staple gun. The antral end, including the previous pyloroplasty, is occluded with a crushing clamp.

50 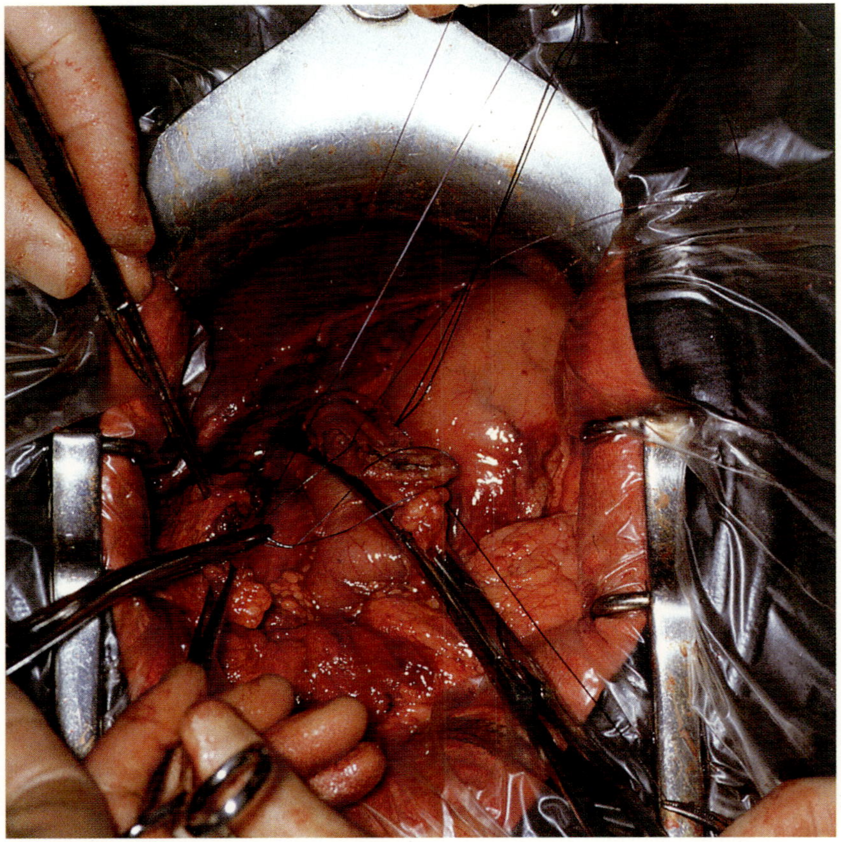

51 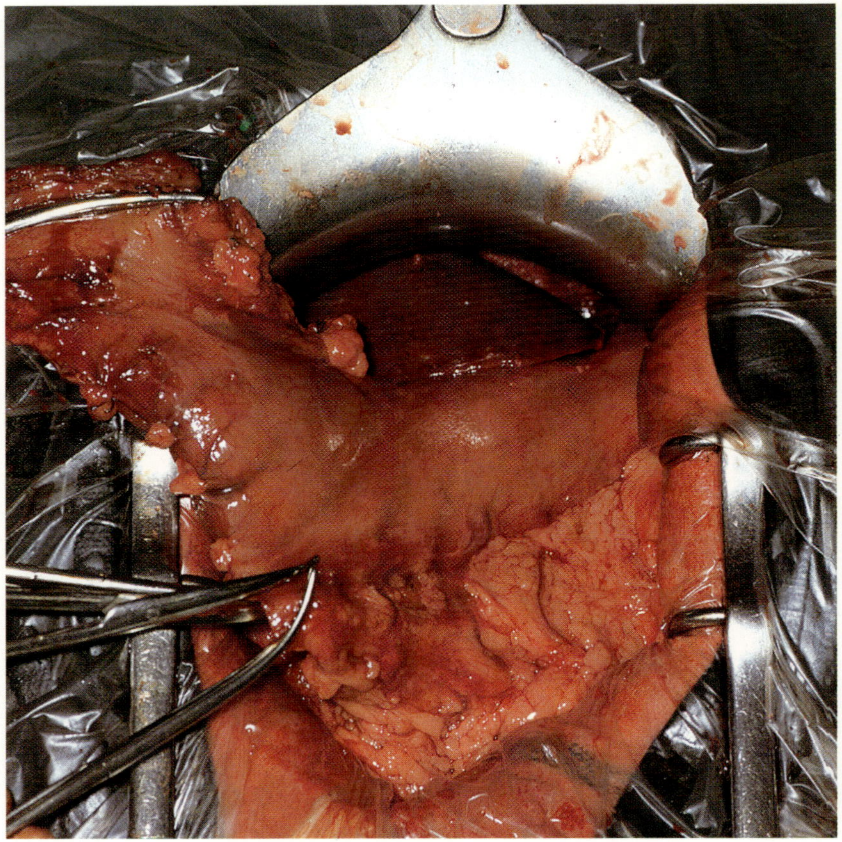

50 An intestinal crushing clamp is placed across the pylorus just proximal to the staple line. The duodenum is divided and the stapled end has the bleeding points coagulated with diathermy and the duodenal stump is buried with a 3/0 vicryl suture.

51 The antrum and part of the body of the stomach has its blood supply divided on both the lesser and the greater curve.

52

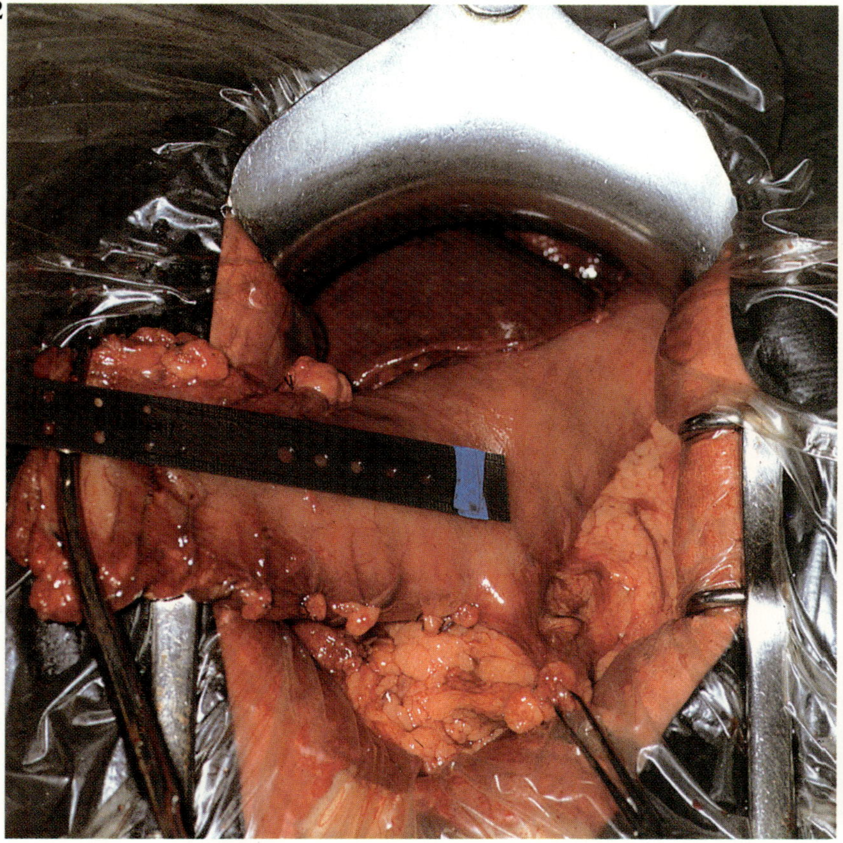

52 This patient, an average-sized male adult, has an intact stomach, so the extent of the antrectomy is measured as 10cm, using a sterile metal rule.

53

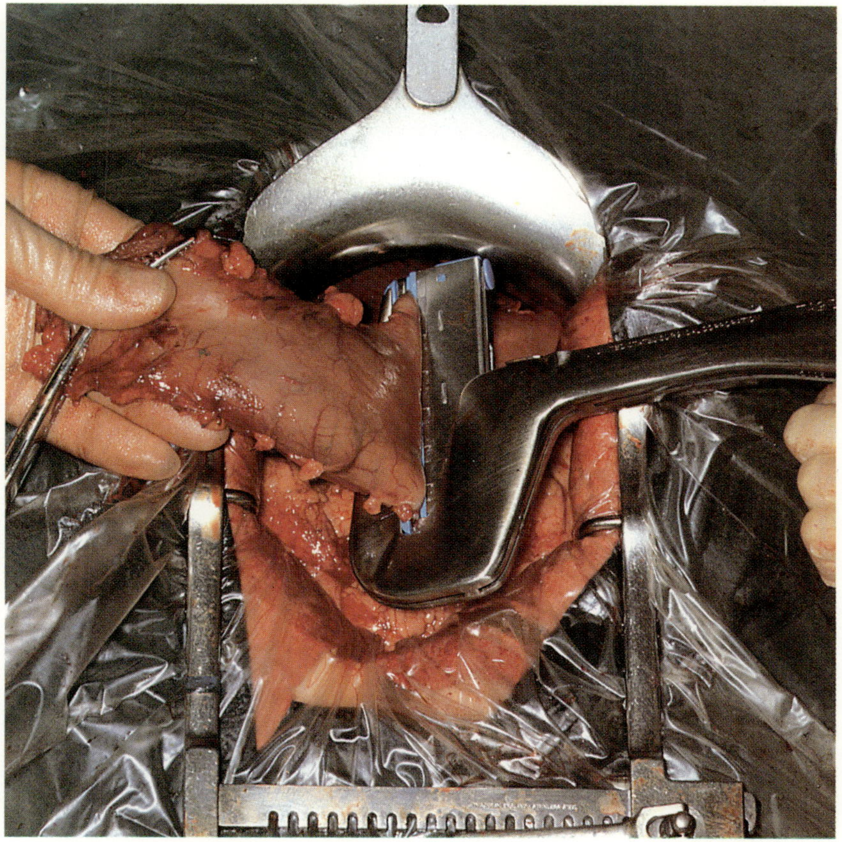

53 At the line of the antral excision, 10cm proximal to the pylorus, a TA 90 staple gun is placed vertically downwards from just proximal to the incisura angularis to the greater curve. The staple gun is fired placing a parallel upper row of staples across the stomach.

54

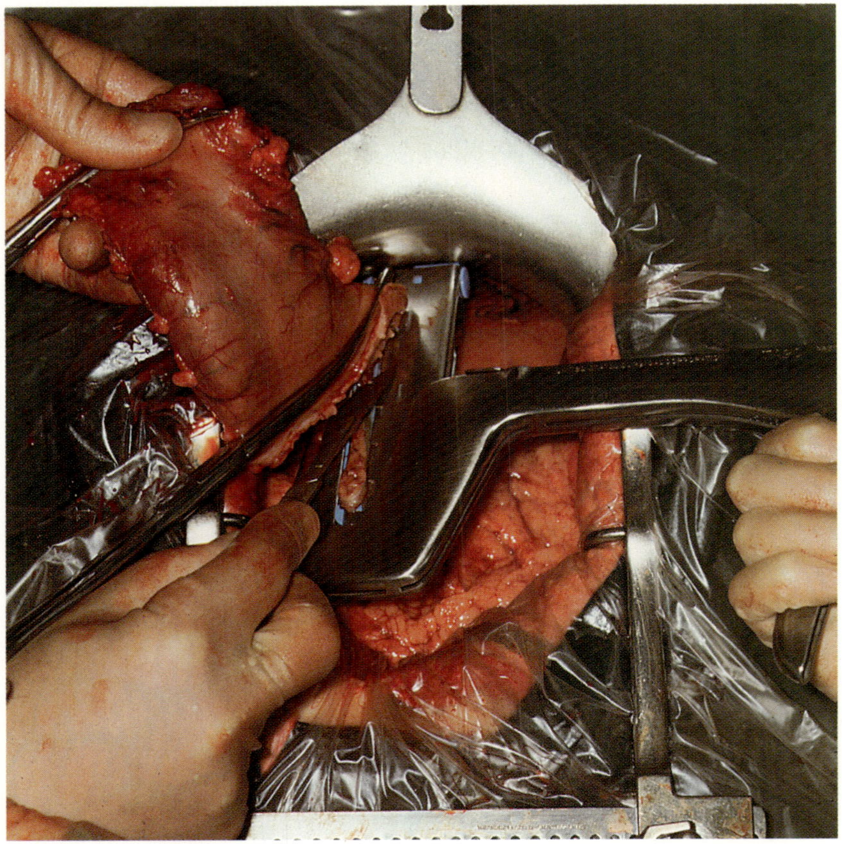

55

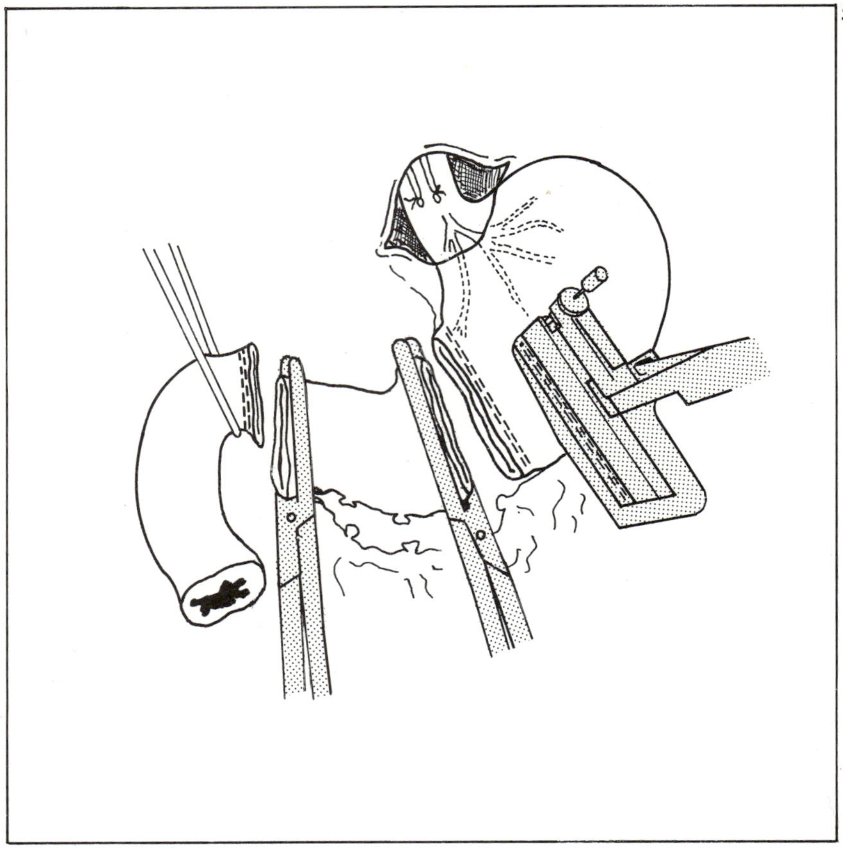

54 Another crushing clamp is placed across the stomach and the stomach is divided just beyond the staple gun.

55 The duodenal stump and the gastric remnant have both been occluded with autosuture staples. The antrum is seen clamped between two crushing intestinal clamps. The vagotomy has been completed.

56
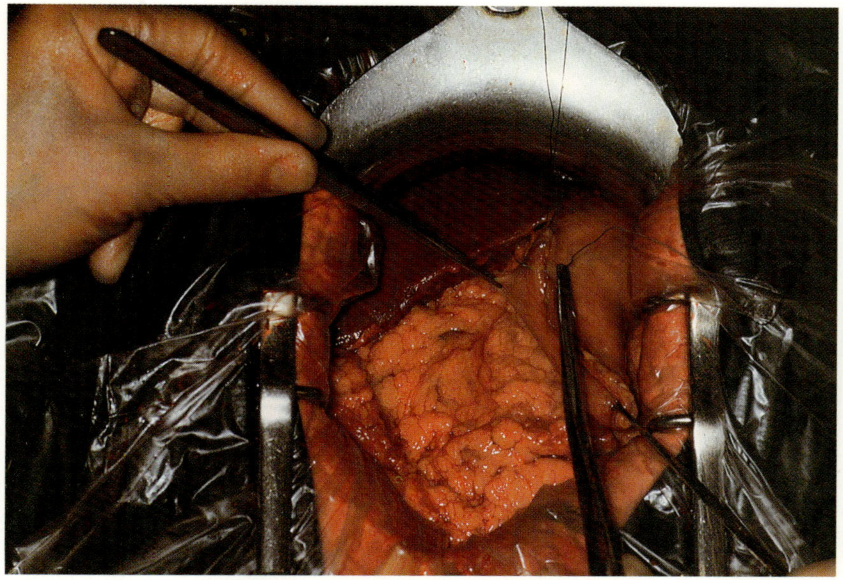

57
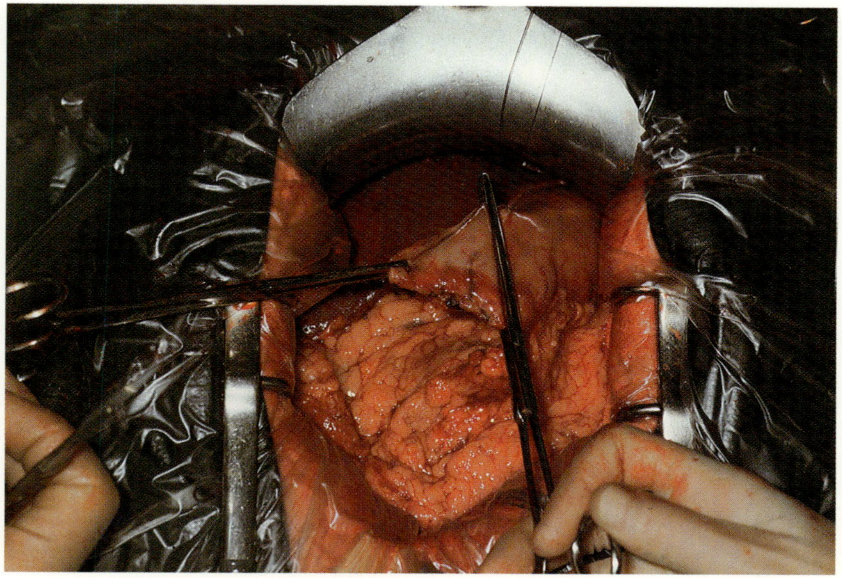

56 The staple line in the stomach has any bleeding points coagulated with diathermy and the lesser curve end of the staple line is oversewn and buried with a 3/0 vicryl suture.

57 and 58 The greater curve end of the proximal stomach remnant that has been closed with the TA 90 stapler is grasped and pulled to the left with tissue forceps. The corner so produced is clamped with a crushing intestinal clamp and the triangular portion removed. The size of the lumen so created is judged to be the same as that of the jejunum to which it will be sutured.

58
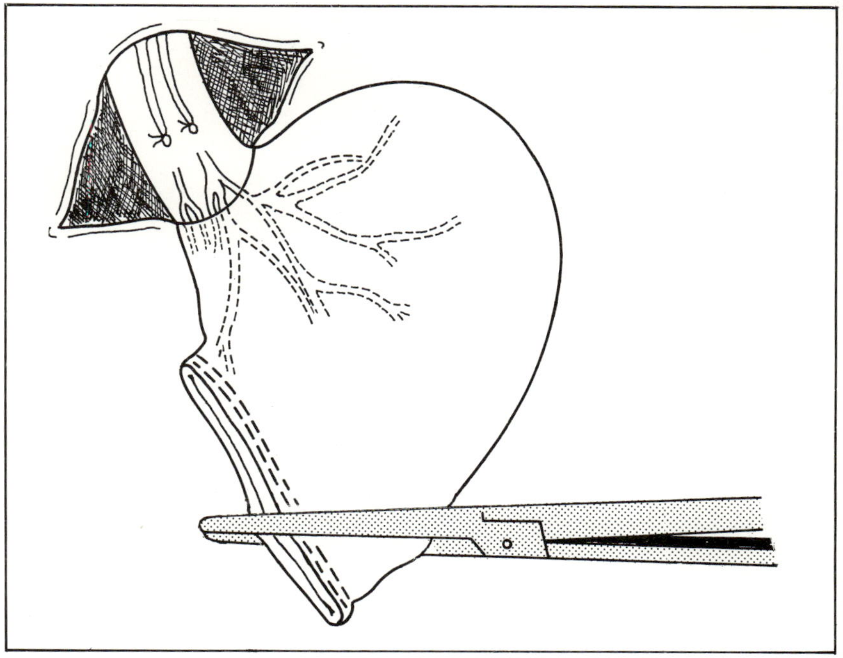

59a

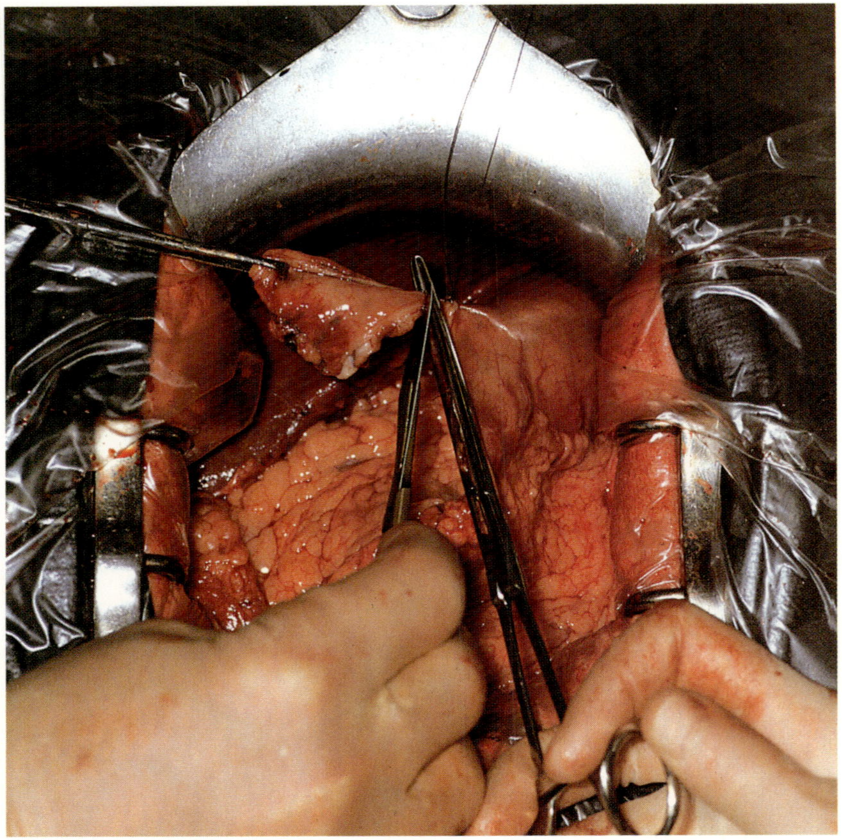

59b

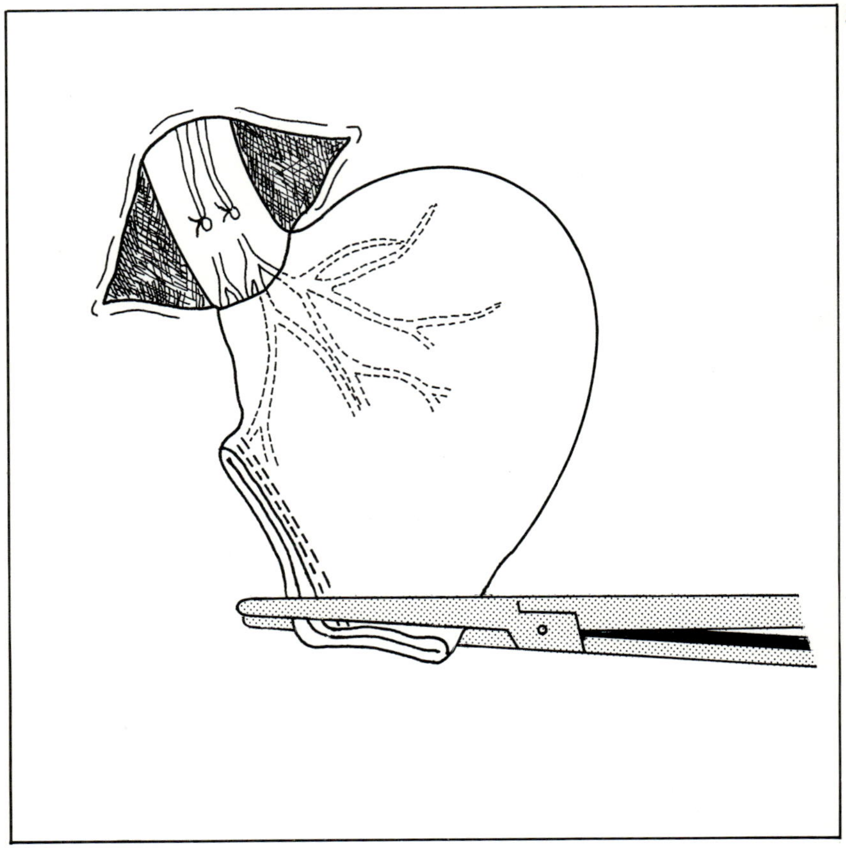

59 (a and b) **The triangular end of the greater curve is cut off with a scalpel blade.**

Creating the Roux loop

60

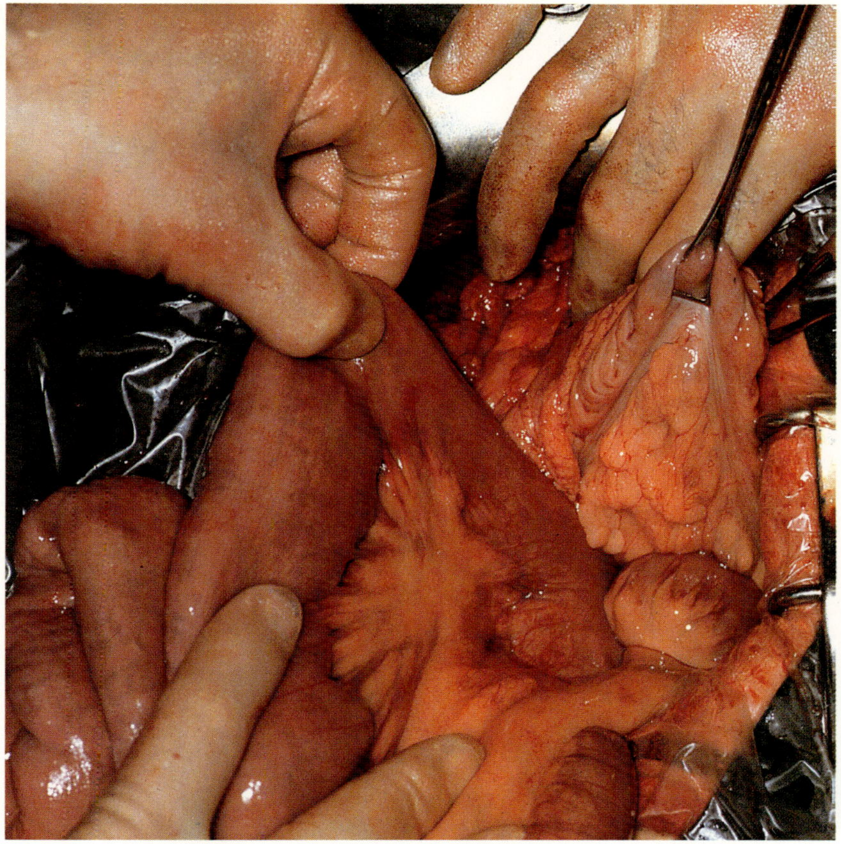

61

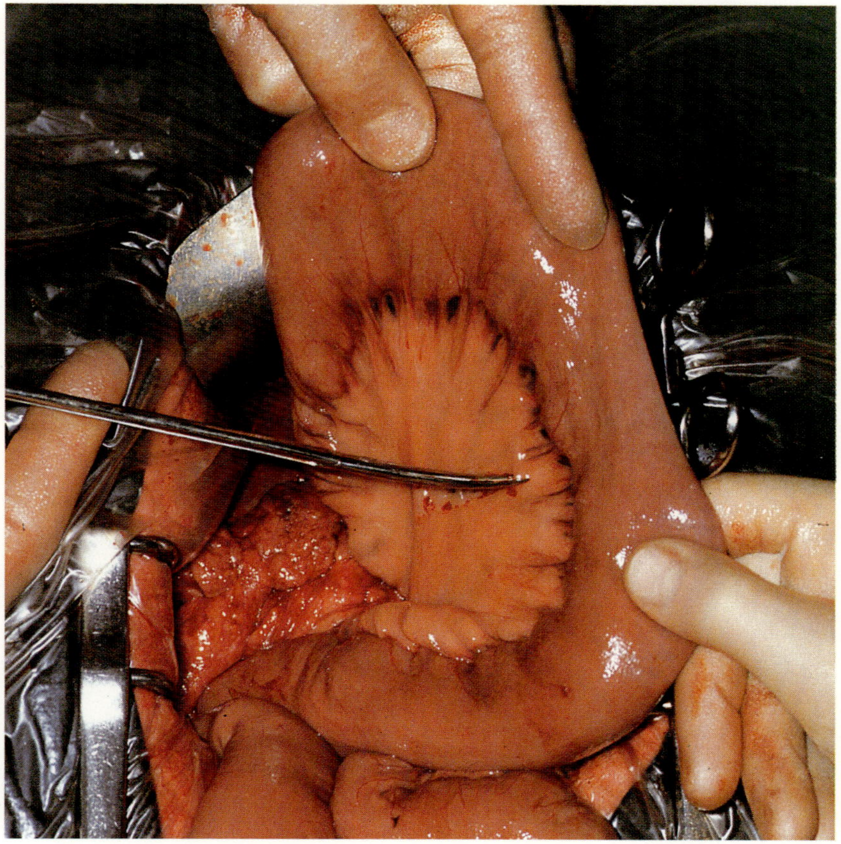

60 Lifting up the mesocolon with non-crushing tissue forceps the duodenojejunal junction is identified and the first loop of jejunum is located. The loop must be sufficiently long to enable the distal end of it to be brought up and anastomosed to the stomach. This point is being grasped by the operator's left hand.

61 The blood vessels forming the vascular arcade of the jejunal loop to be divided are then identified.

62

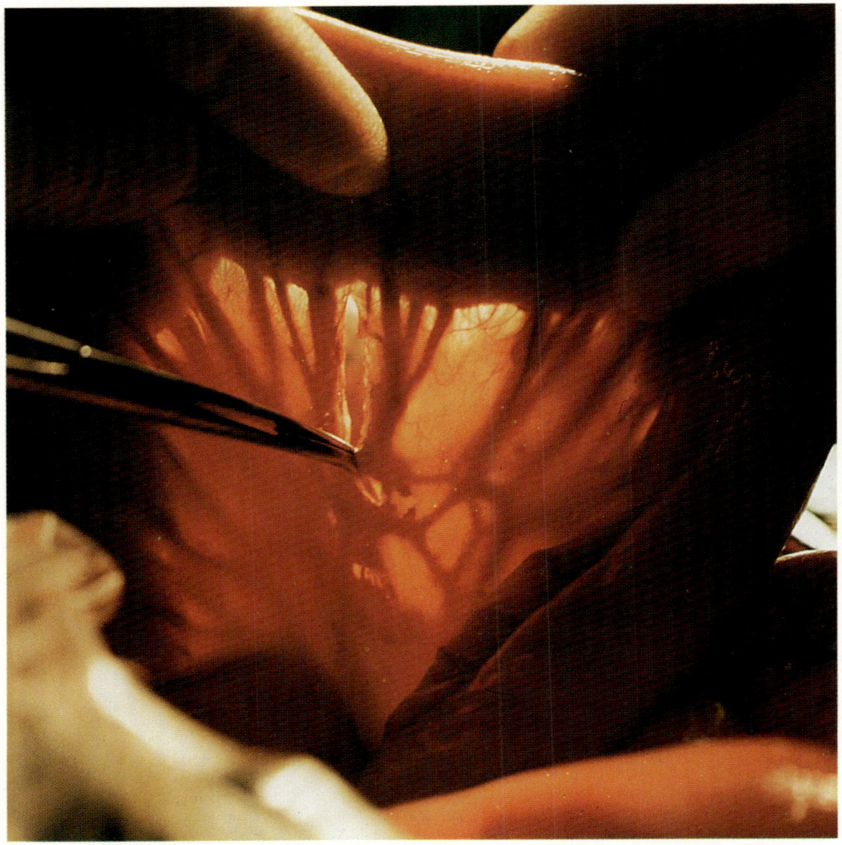

62 **In the fat patient the identification of vascular arcade is facilitated by transilluminating the mesentery of the gut with a light behind it. This enables the blood vessels to be seen quite clearly.** They are then divided and ligated using fine arterial forceps and 3/0 vicryl ligatures.

63

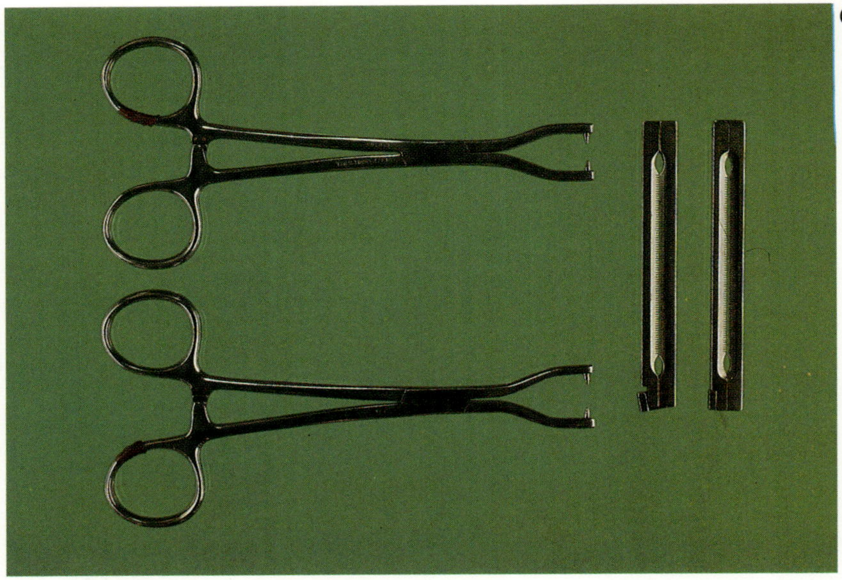

63 **Soft non-crushing intestinal clamps, which are a modification of Pott's arterial clamps, having been designed to be used with detachable handles.** These clamps enable the divided loop of gut to be brought up through the small hole in the mesocolon.

64

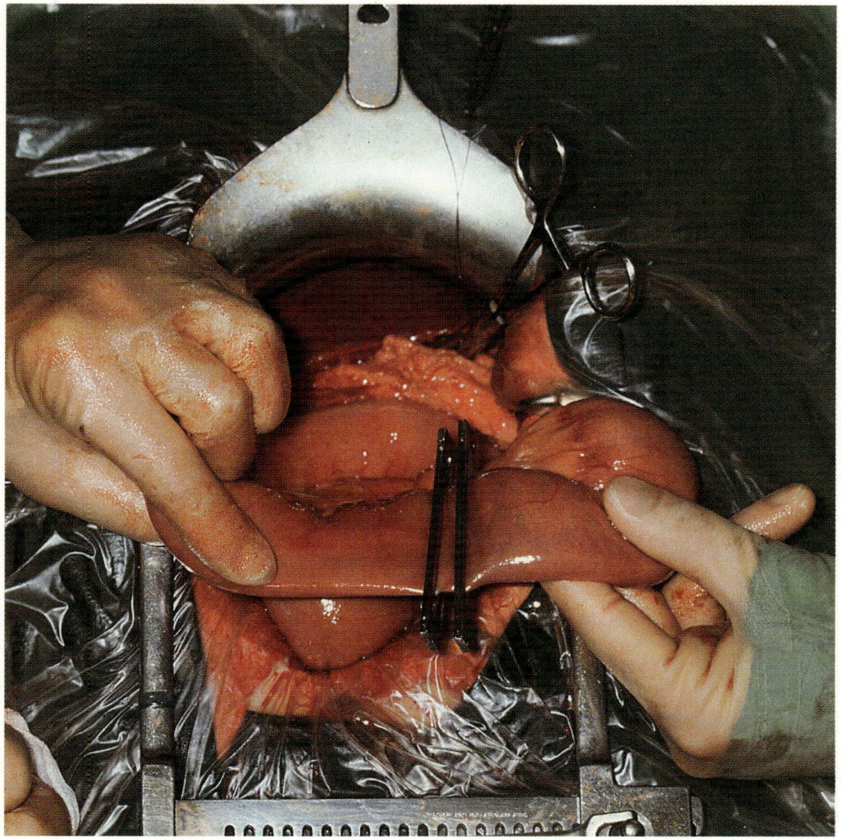

65

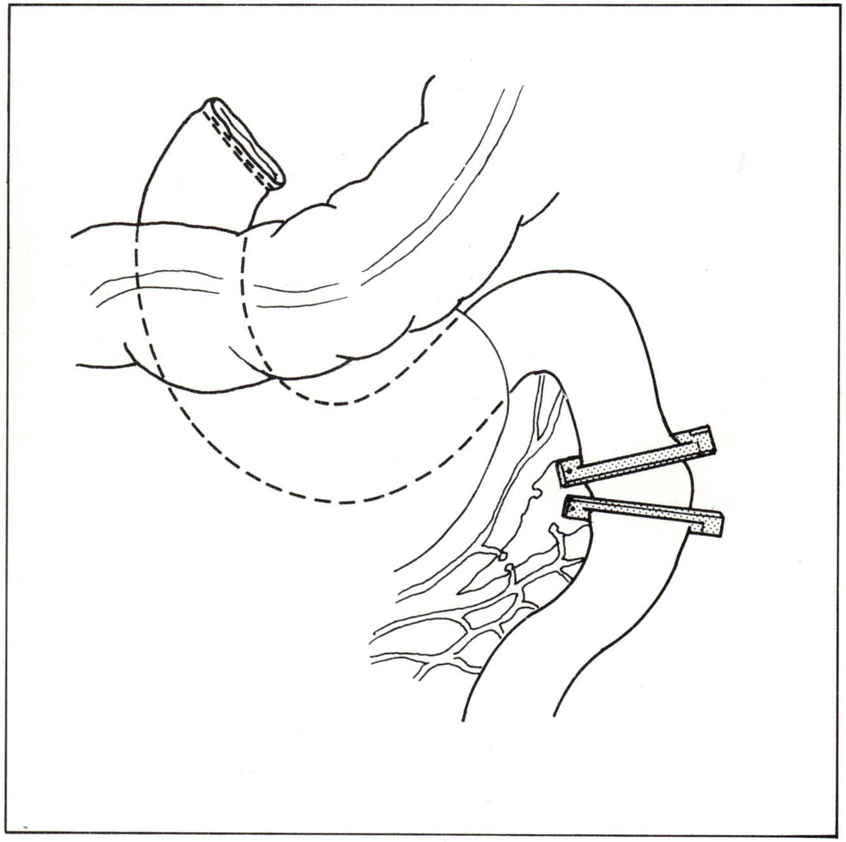

64 and 65 Two Pace-Pott's handleless clamps are placed across the apex of the mobilised proximal jejunal loop.

66

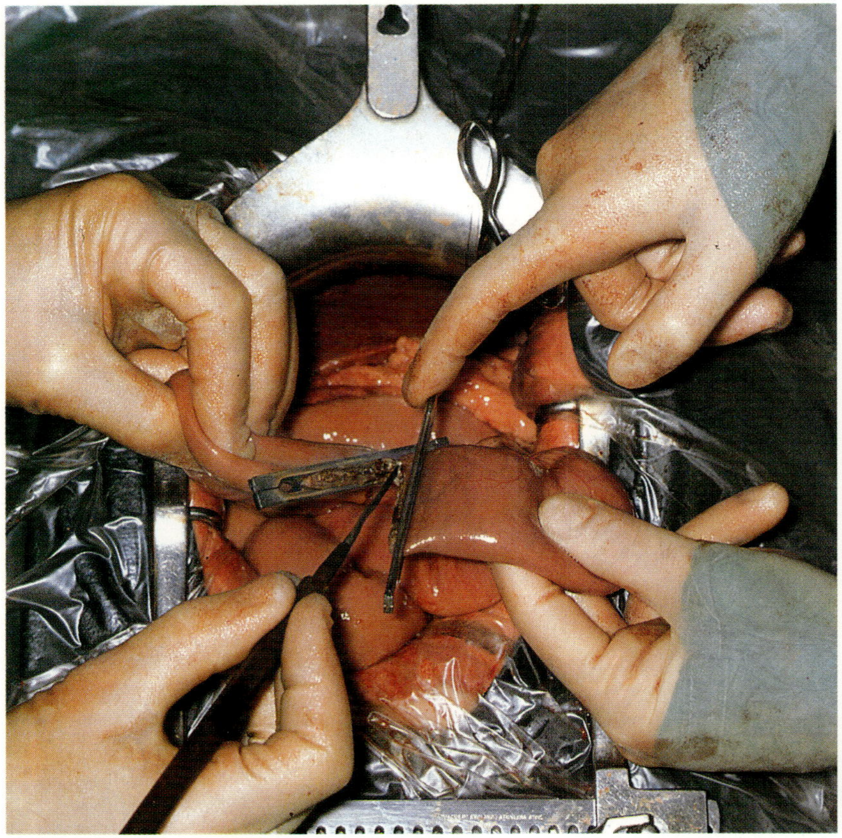

66 The jejunum is divided between the clamps using a cutting diathermy current.

67

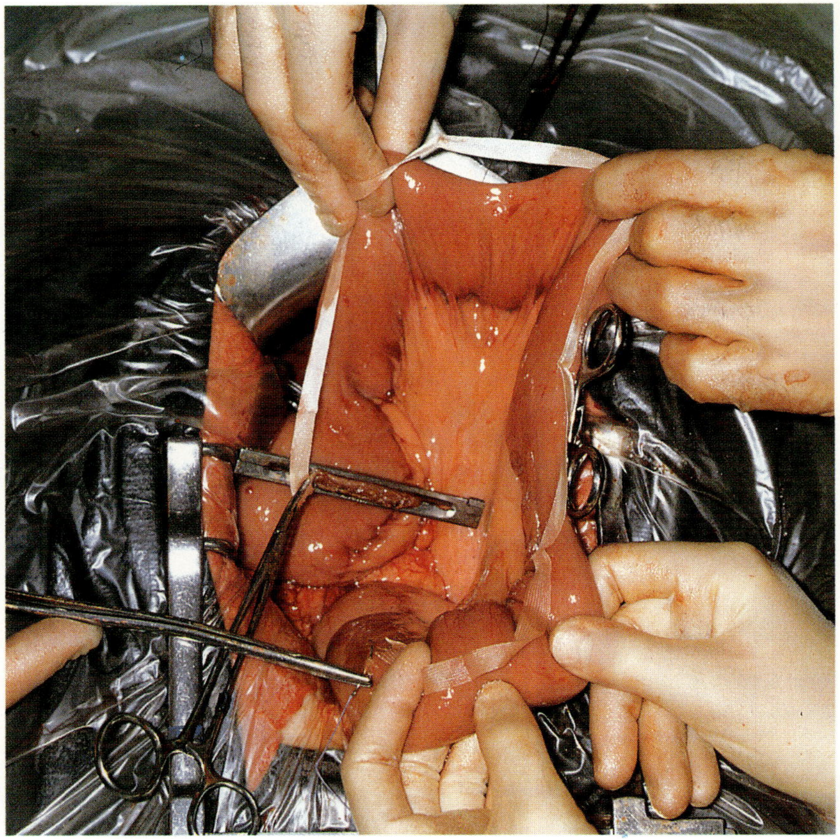

67 To facilitate the measurement of a 60 cm loop for the Roux-en-y anastomosis a measured tape is prepared and laid around the edge of the bowel. The point 60 cm distal to the Pace-Pott's clamp is marked with a stay suture for later identification.

68

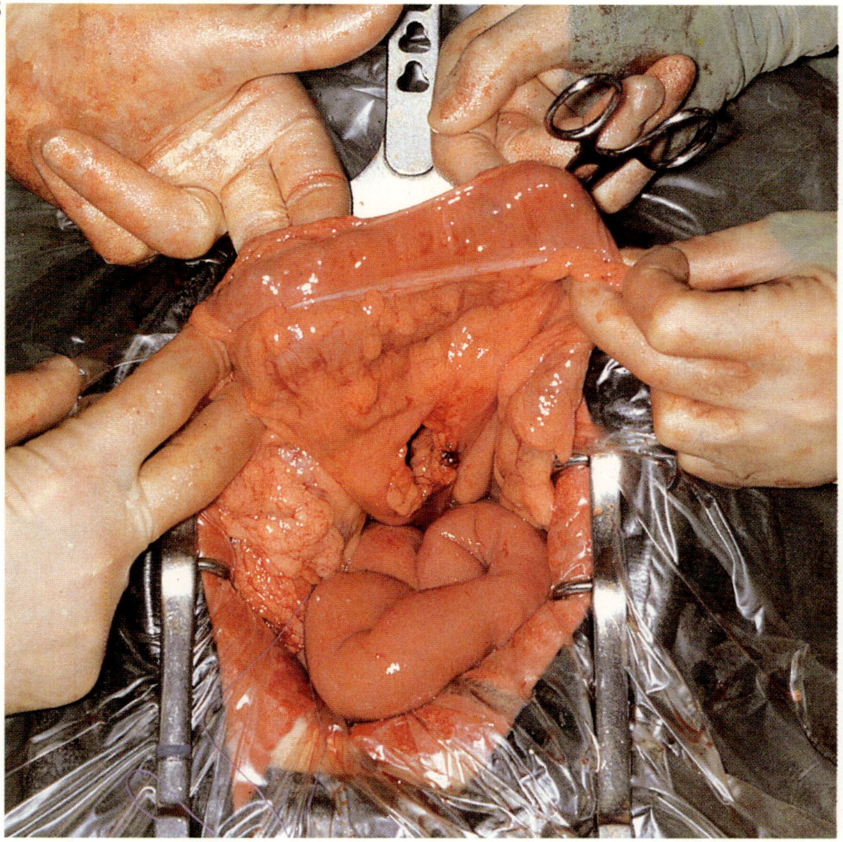

69

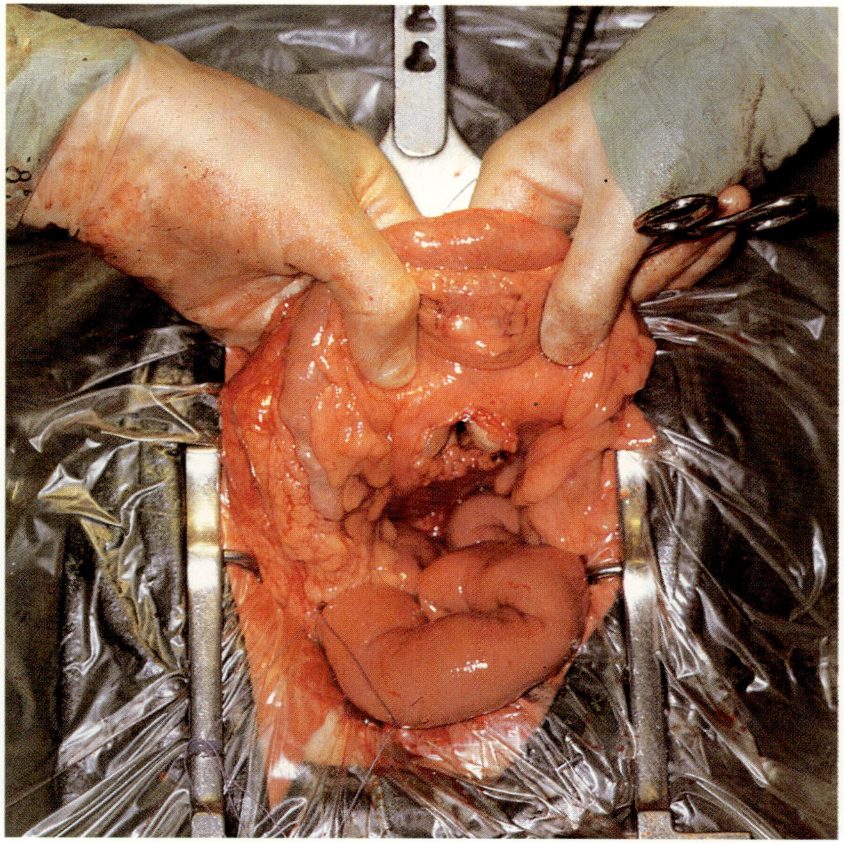

68 The mesocolon is then lifted up by the surgeon and the assistant and an avascular 'window' is found in it.

69 A hole is made in the mesocolon and the Pace-Pott's clamp, attached to the distal part of the divided jejunal loop is brought up through the hole in the mesocolon to be anastomosed end-to-end to the gastric remnant.

70

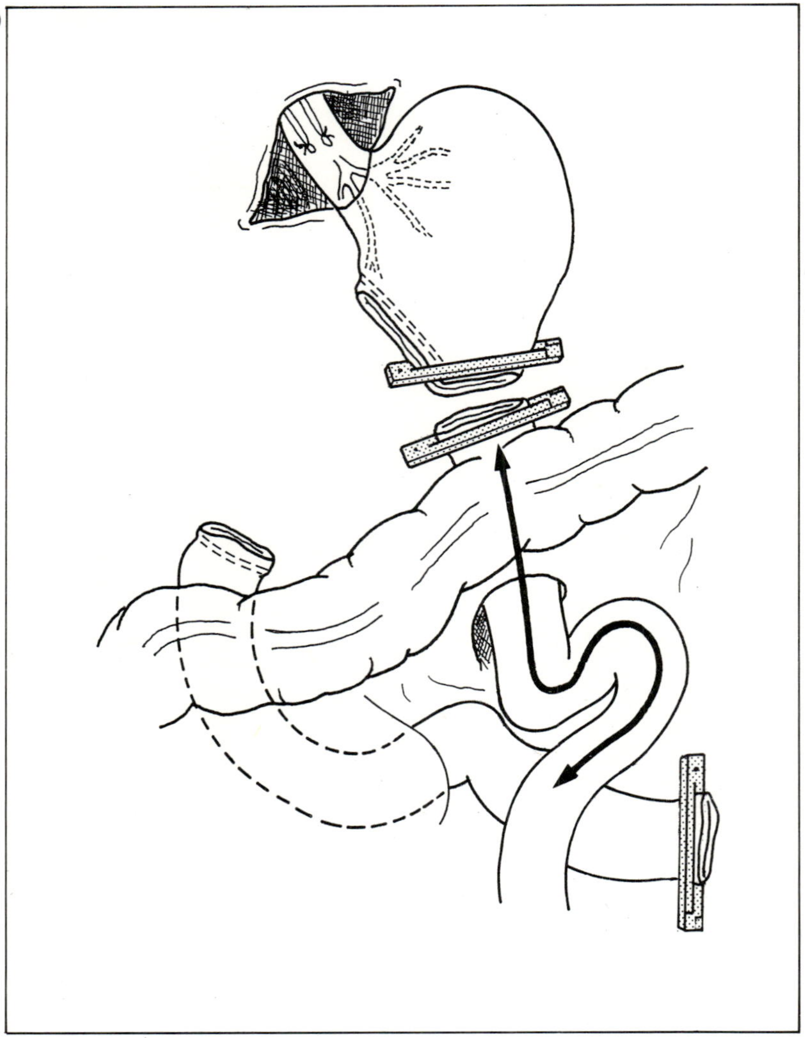

71

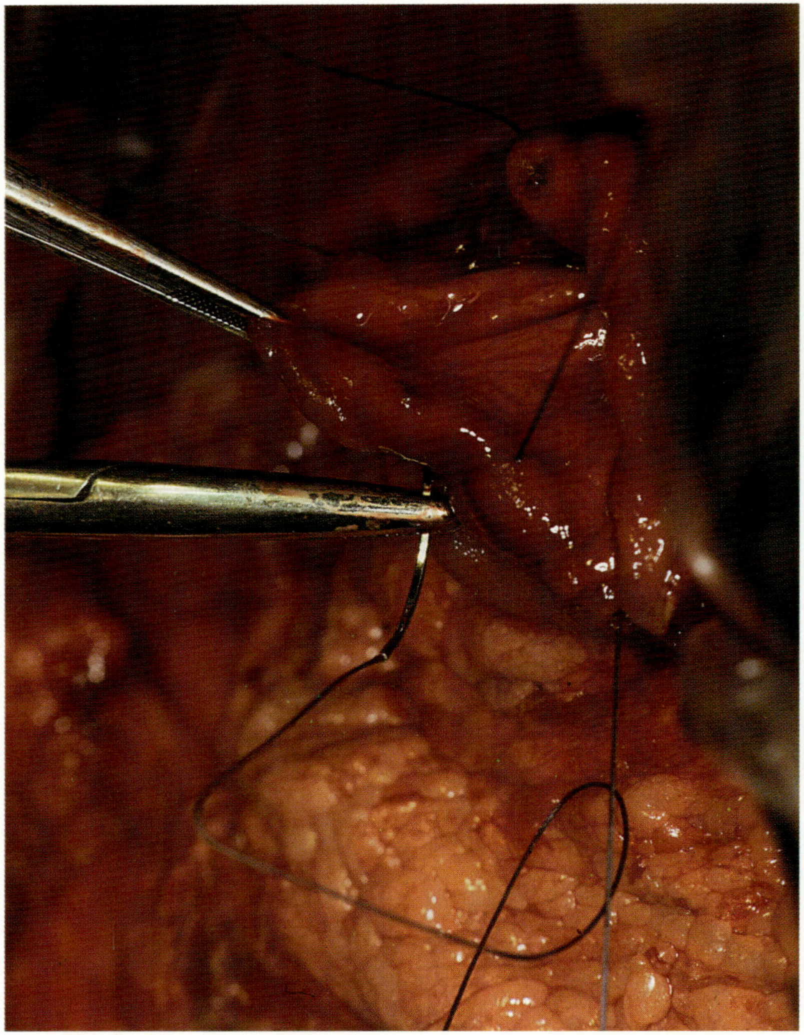

70 An anastomosis is performed between the similar sized lumina of the amputated greater-curve end of the gastric remnant and the end of jejunum. The anastomosis is conveniently and safely performed by placing stay sutures of 3/0 vicryl at either end and in the centre; then running a continuous 3/0 vicryl suture across the posterior layer.

71 The cut end of the greater curve of the gastric remnant is sutured to the distal end of the jejunal loop. A posterior layer of continuous sutures has been placed.

72

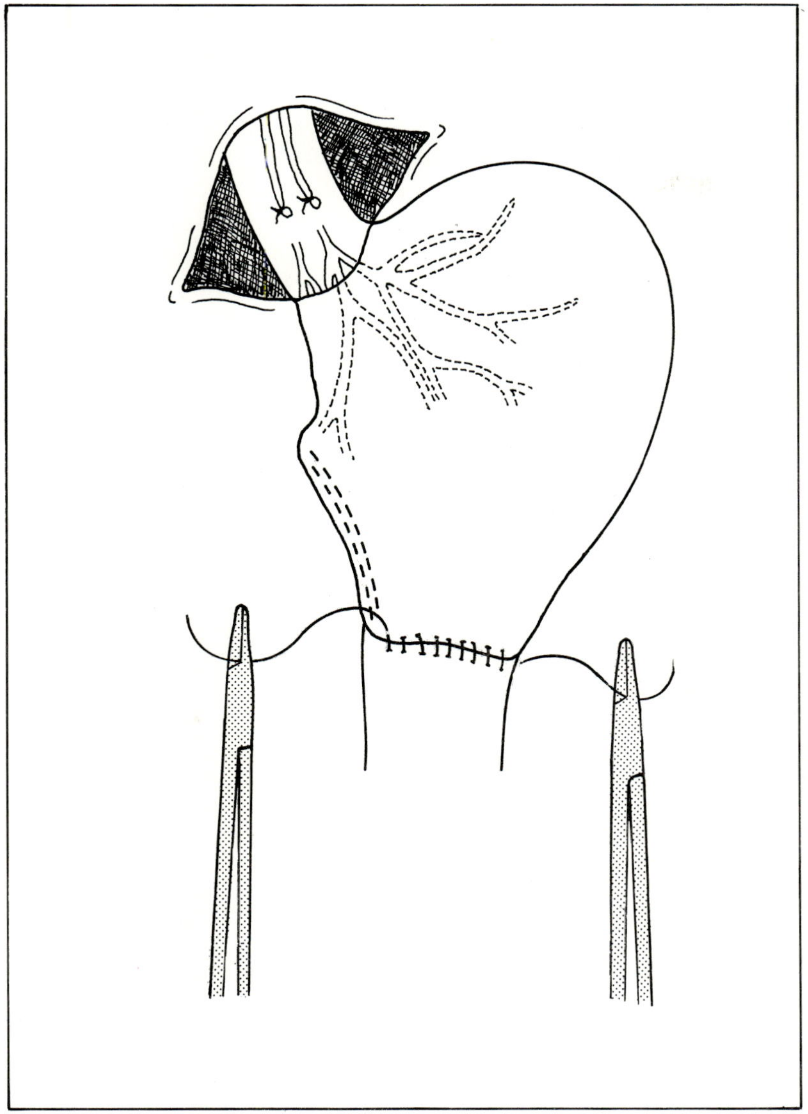

72 **The anterior layer of the anastomosis is closed in a similar manner, using an over-and-over suture with edge-to-edge apposition.** It errs, if at all, in the direction of slight inversion of the suture line.

73

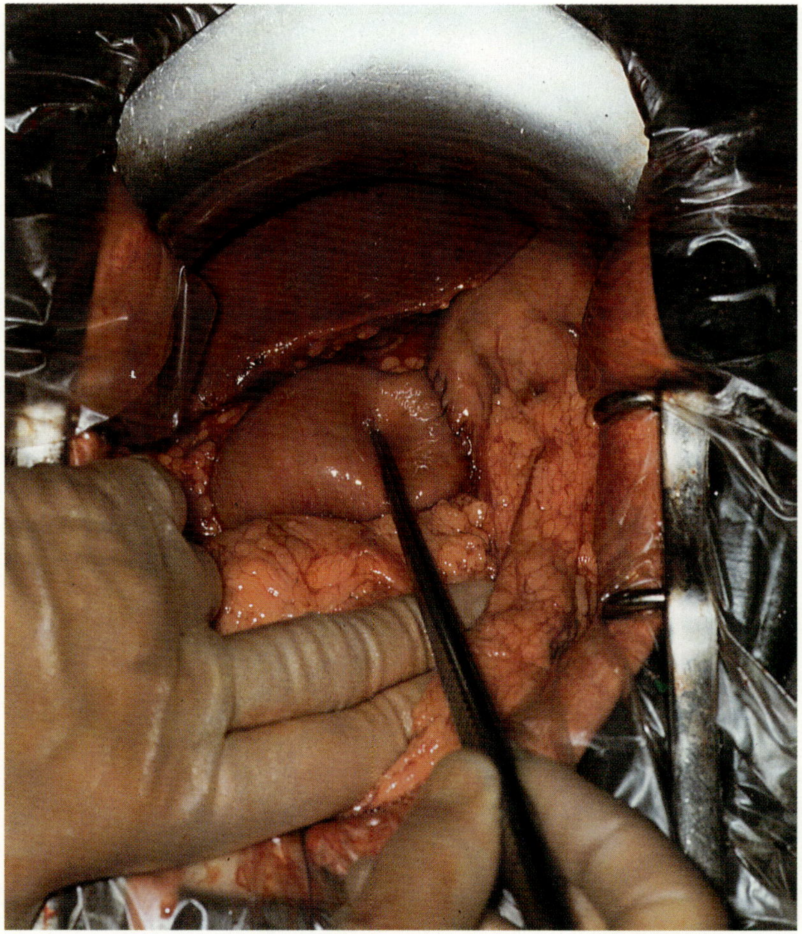

73 **The completed anastomosis between the jejunal loop and the stomach.** The difference in colour is always easily appreciated; the stomach is paler and pinker and the jejunum slightly brown.

74

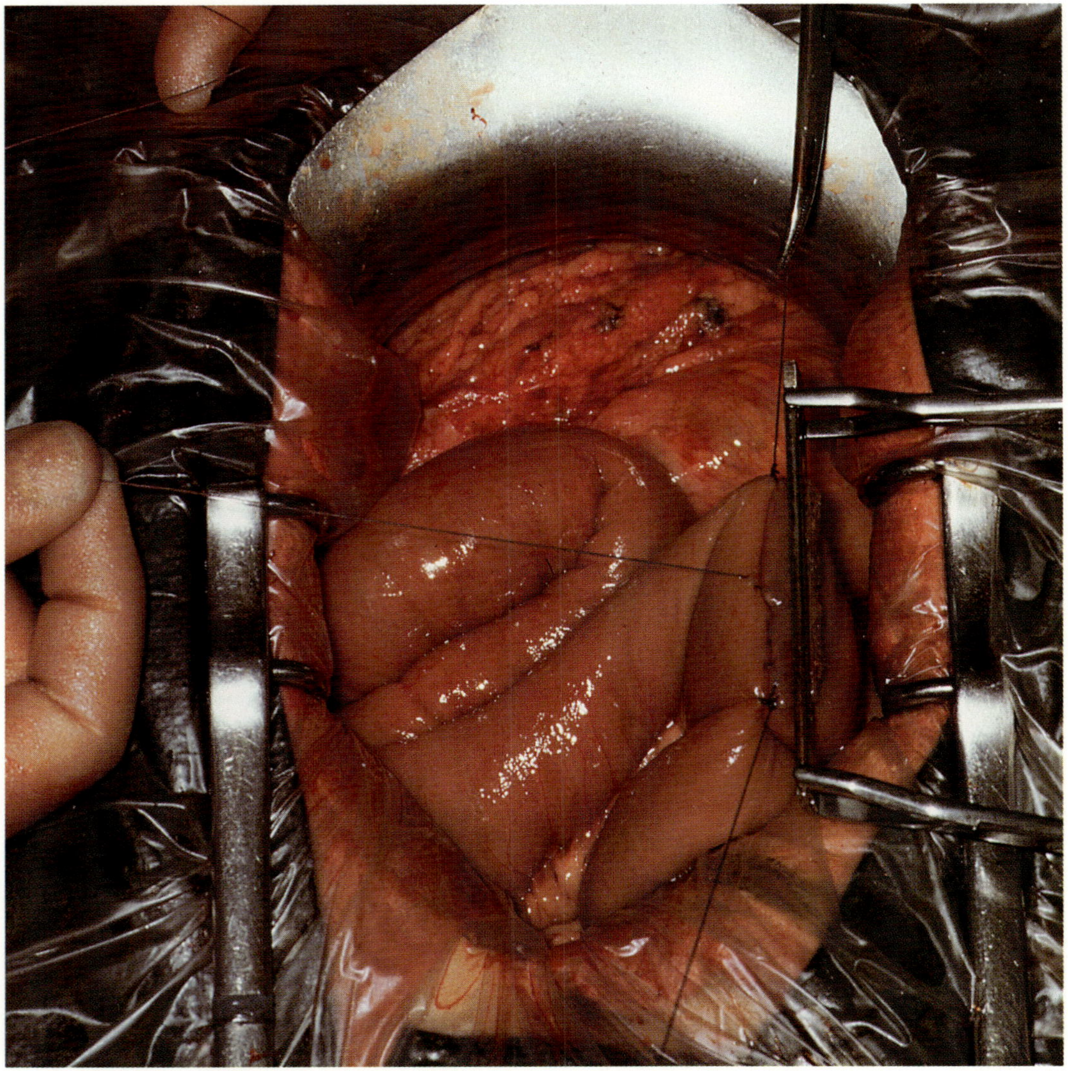

74 The previously marked loop of jejunum, 60 cm 'down stream', is brought up and sutured to the proximal end of the first jejunal loop. This has been included by a Pace-Pott's clamp. Sutures are placed at either end and in the centre of the cut edge of jejunal loop.

75 A diathermy cutting current is used to open the lumen of the distal jejunum.

75
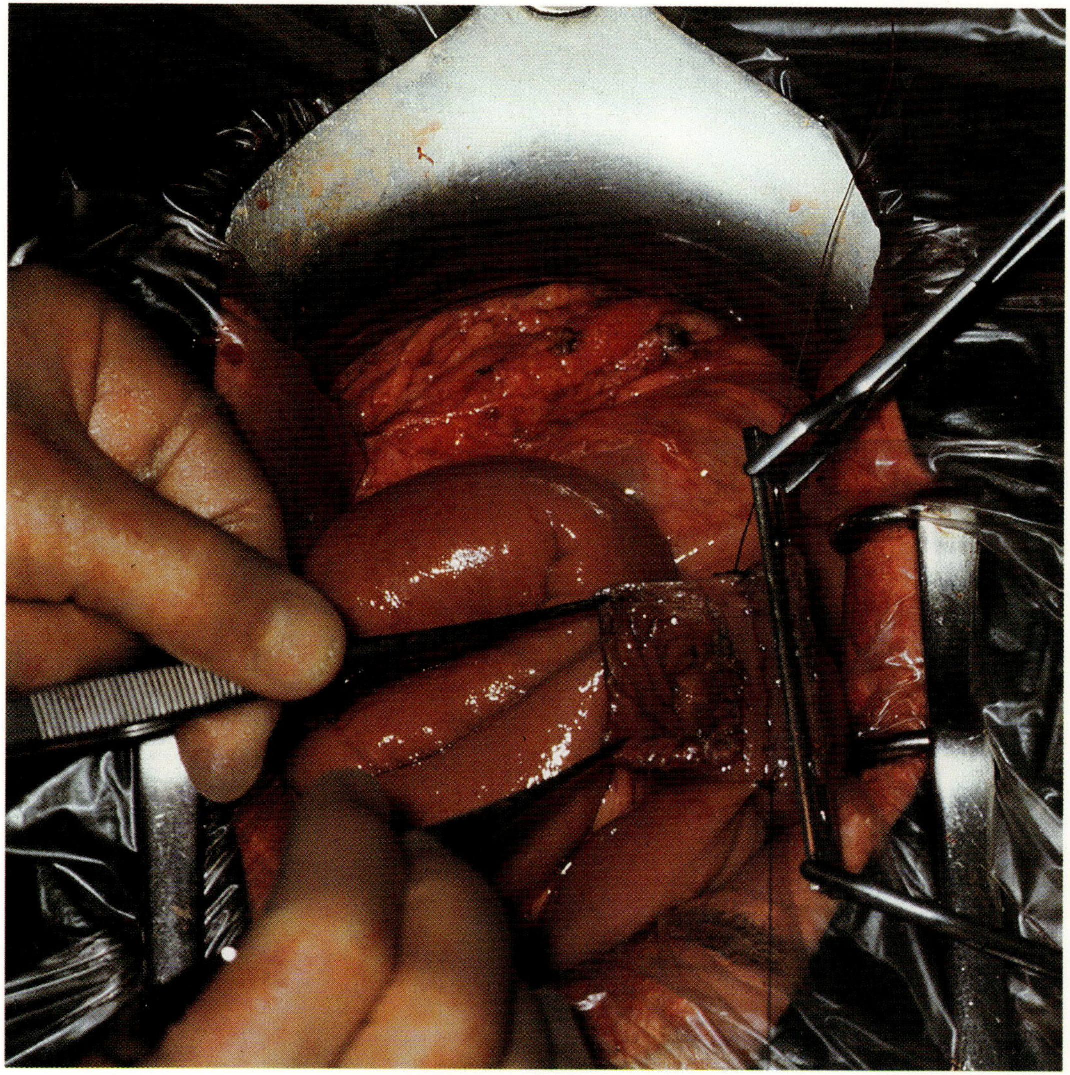

76

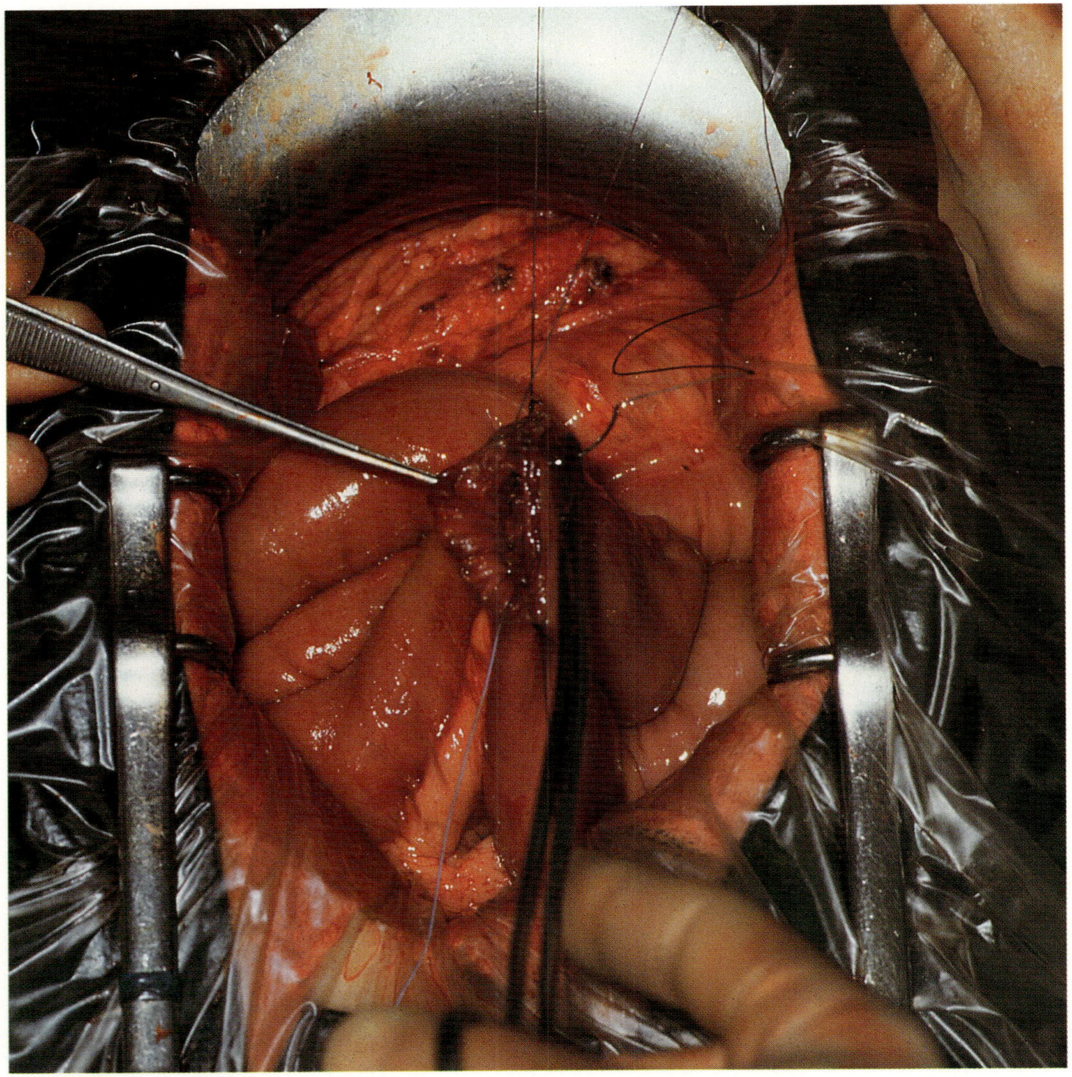

76 The Pace-Pott's clamp is removed and the cut edges of the bowel are anastomosed end-to-side using continuous 3/0 vicryl. The anterior layer of the anastomosis is completed similarly.

Anastomosis completed

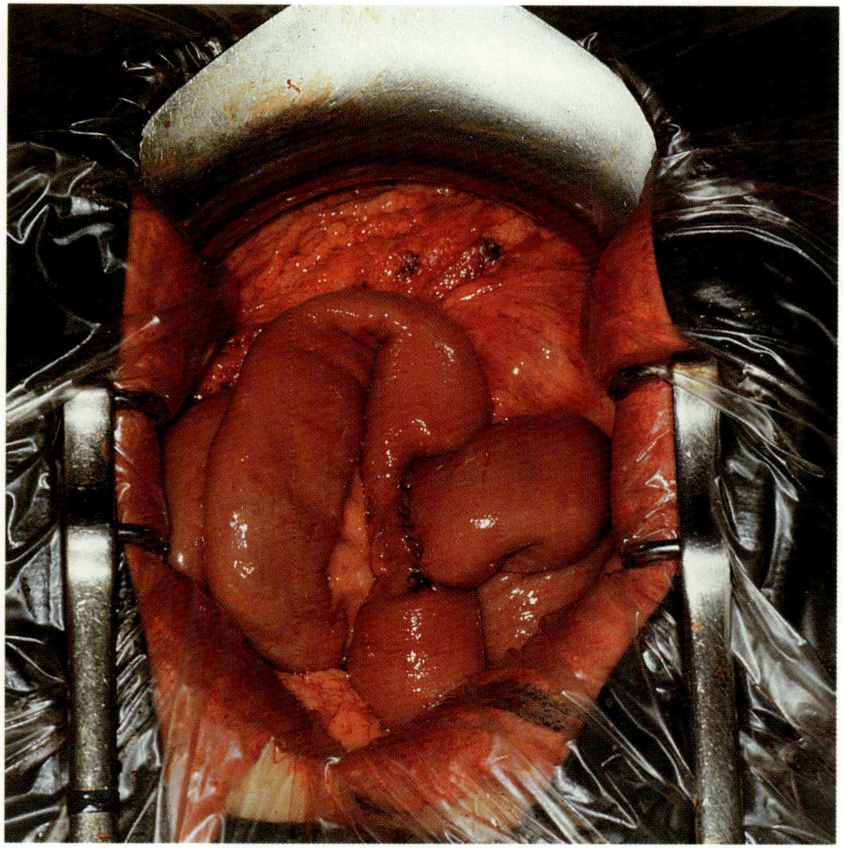

77 A continuous suture of the serosal layer is then continued around the front of the anastomosis. The hole in the mesocolon is then closed.

78

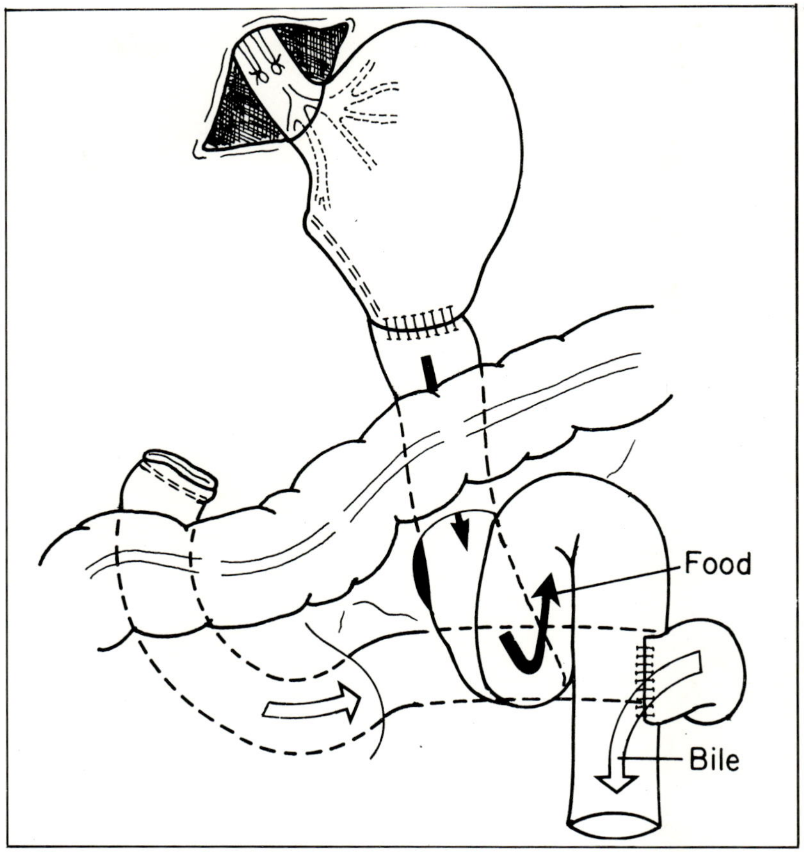

78 The completed anastomosis showing the end-to-end gastro-jejunostomy, the 60 cm retrocolic loop and the end-to-side jejuno-jejunostomy.

79

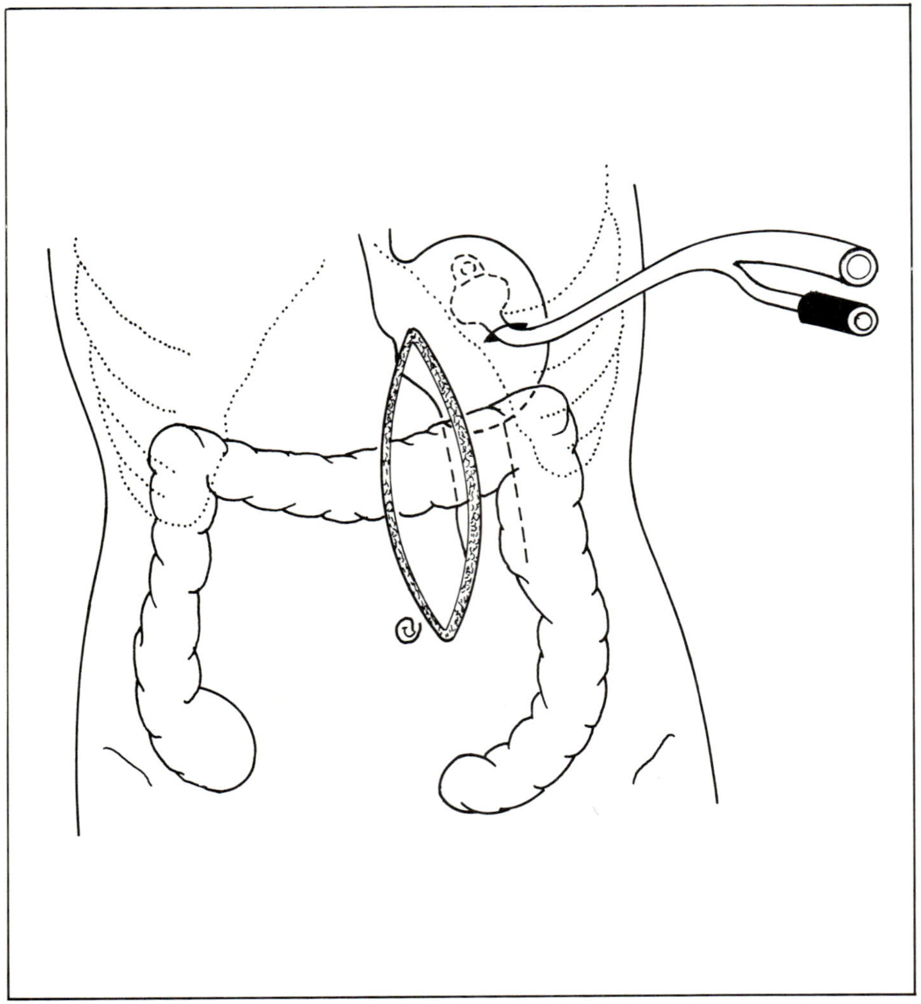

79 A balloon catheter gastrostomy. A gastrostomy drainage of the gastric remnant is offered to those patients in whom some delay in gastric emptying is expected or who have a particular abhorrence of any form of nasogastric intubation. Most accept and welcome it.

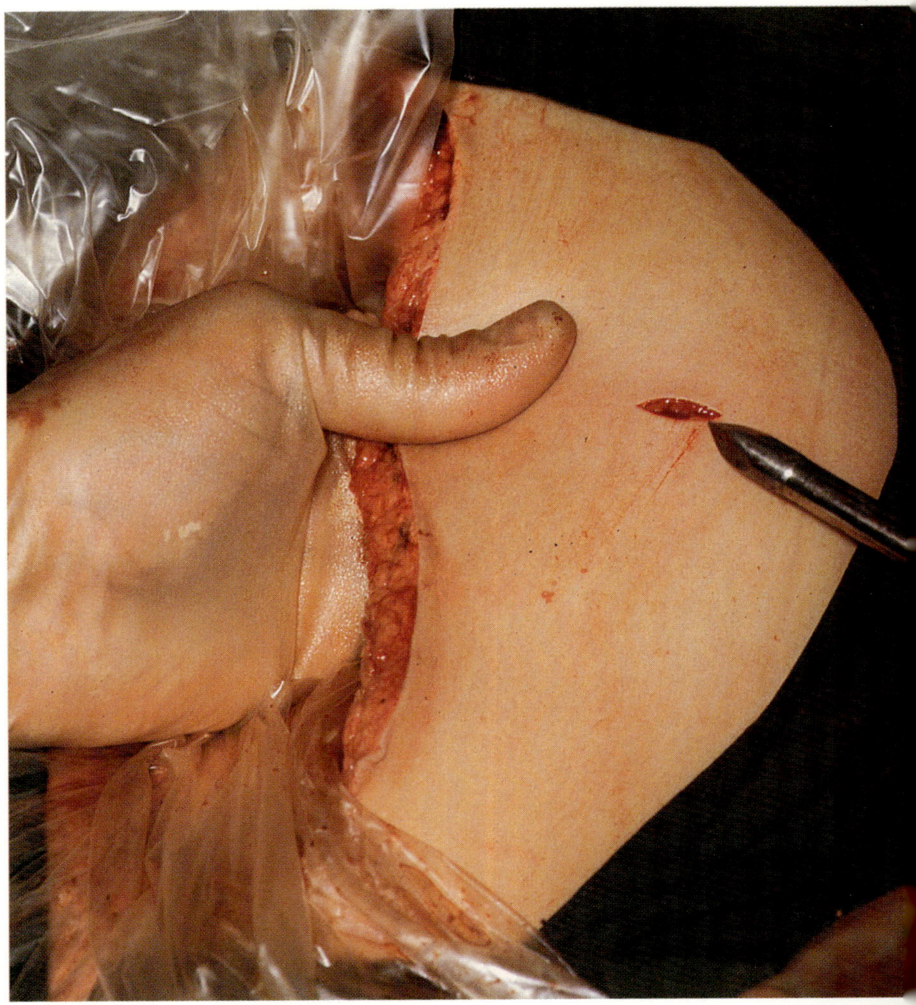

80 A small 'stab' incision is made in the left upper quadrant, a little away from the costal margin. A large cannula, of the type used for draining chests or large hydrocoeles has been modified by removing the flange so that, once the cannula is inserted through the abdominal wall, it can be drawn in or out.

81

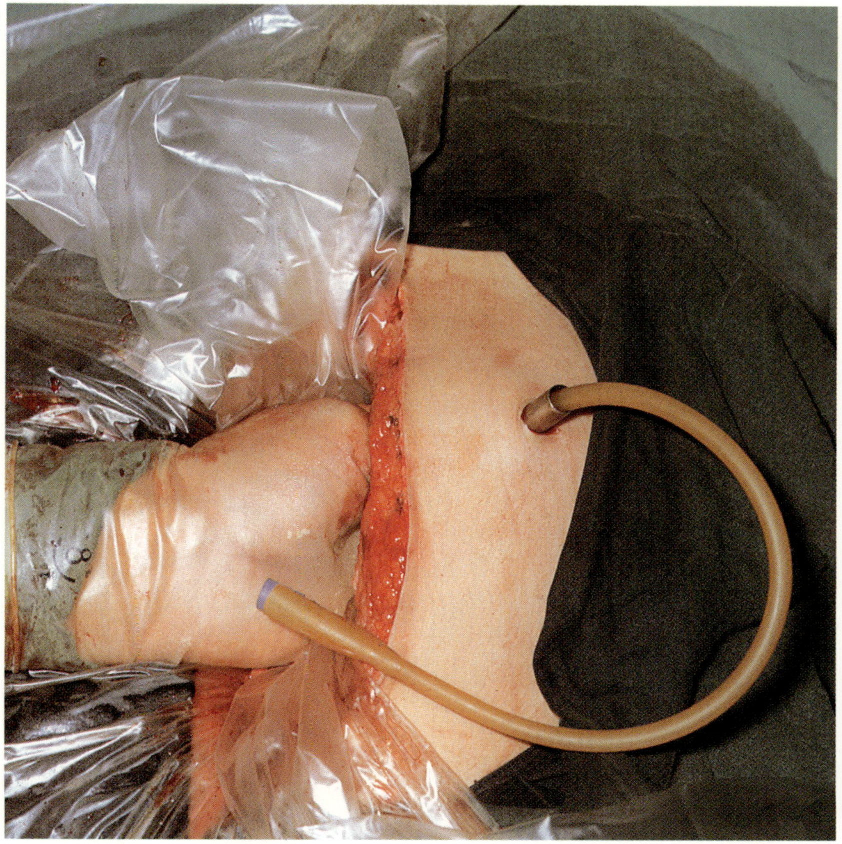

81 The special cannula without the flange is thrust through the abdominal wall, through the small skin incision.

82

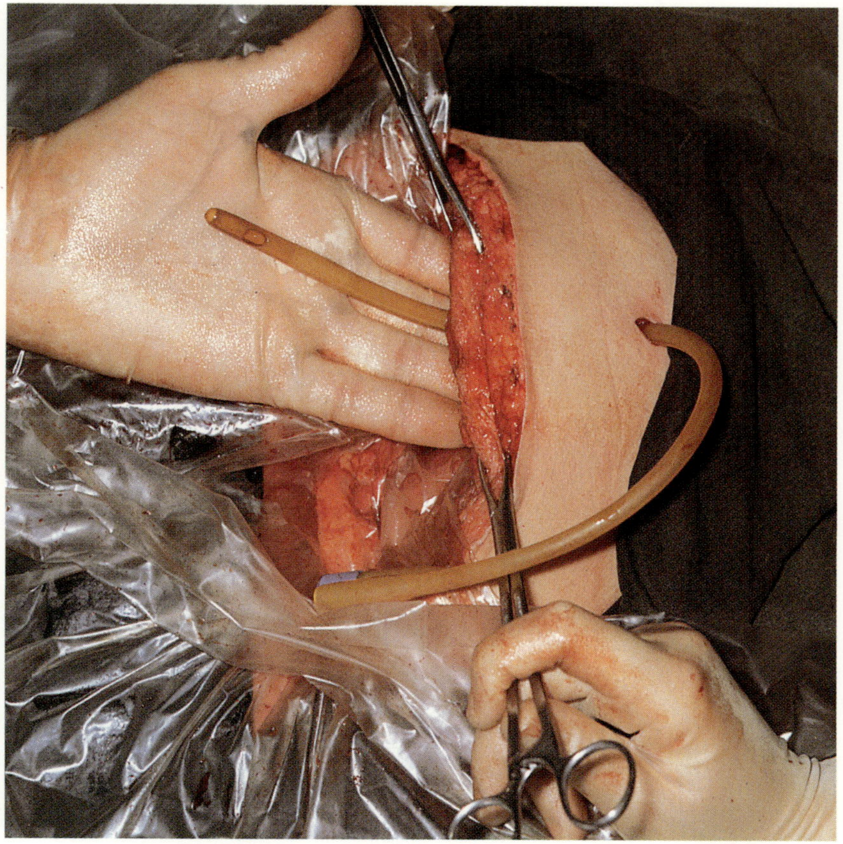

82 A balloon catheter has been placed within the lumen of the cannula. As the cannula is drawn into the inside of the abdomen, the catheter is taken with it.

83

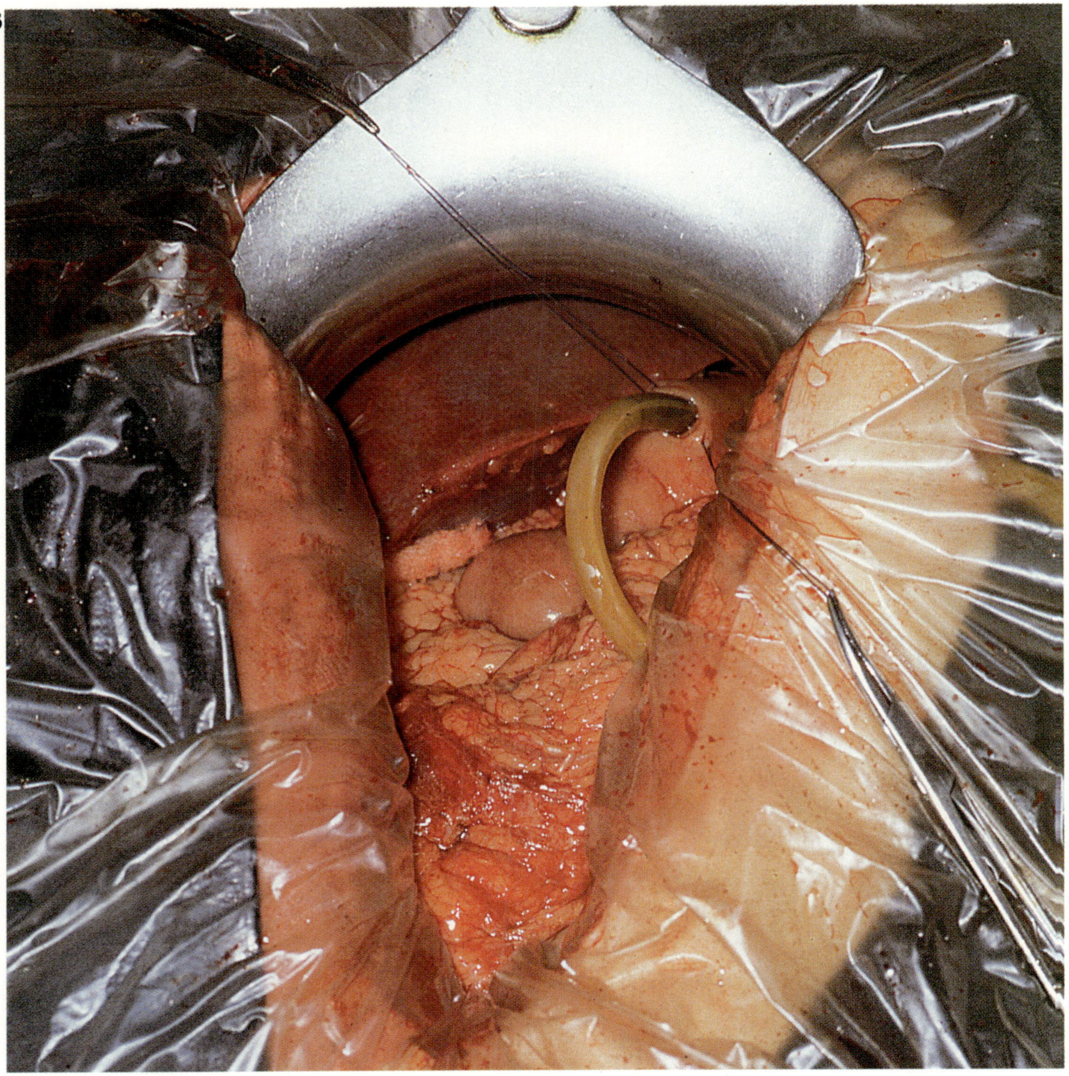

83 A portion of the gastric remnant is selected that can be brought down to the anterior abdominal wall at the site of entry of the catheter. This point on the stomach wall is secured with a stay suture and a hole is made in the stomach with diathermy to allow the tip of the balloon catheter to be passed into the stomach. The balloon is inflated and the hole in the gastric wall is closed securely with two concentric inverting purse-string sutures of catgut.

84 Sutures applied to the gastric wall at the gastrostomy site are used to anchor the stomach to the posterior aspect of the anterior wall. Any greater omentum that can be mobilised is brought up to wrap around this junction for additional safety.

This view is of the back of the anterior abdominal wall showing the use of some adjacent omentum to help to ensure a good seal at the gastrostomy site.

84

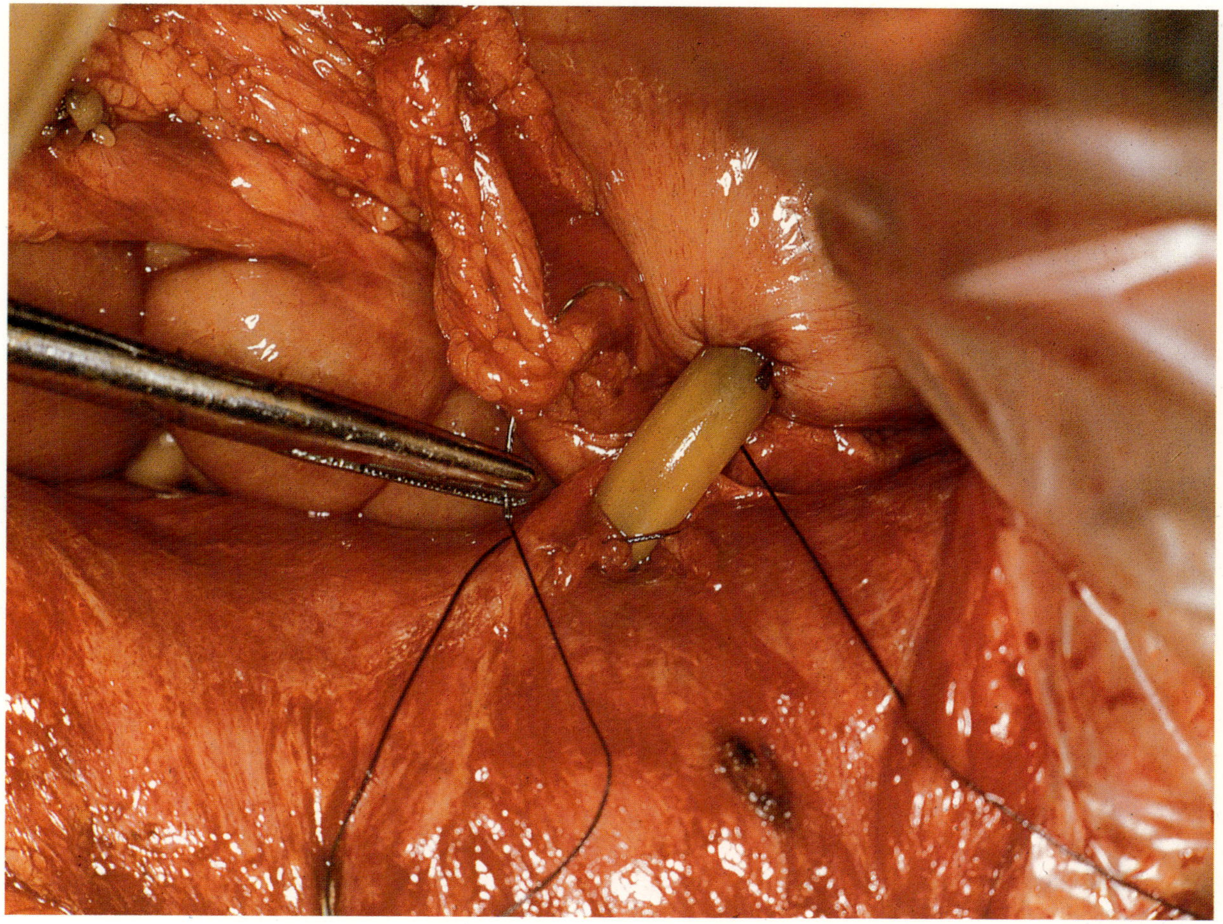

85

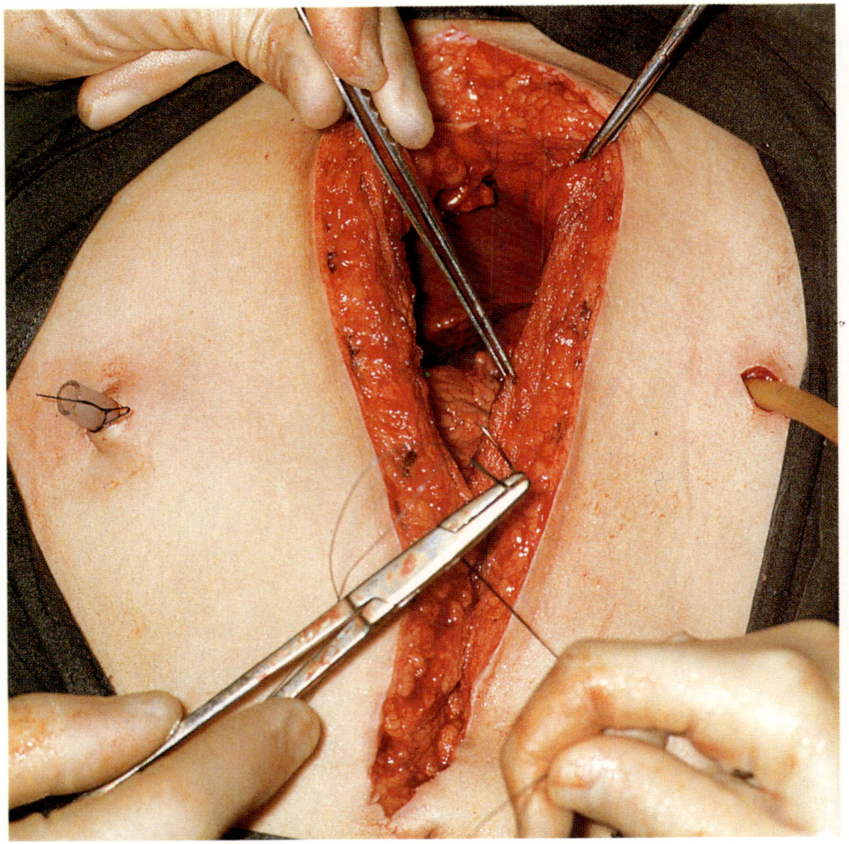

86

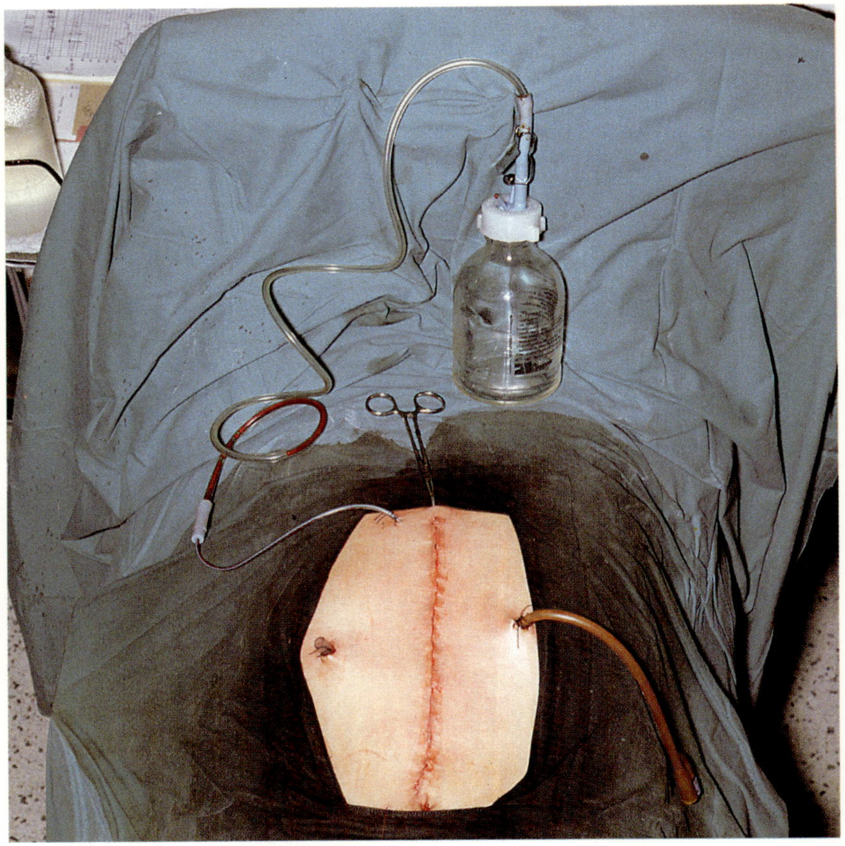

85 A drainage tube has been placed through the right side of the abdomen to drain the duodenal stump and under surface of the liver. The abdomen is being closed with continuous large-bite non-absorbable suture material. **A patient who has achlorhydria and therefore a heavily infected stomach is particularly likely to develop wound infection.** The strength of a continuous loop nylon suture is appreciated. In this patient the fat layer was drained with a small-bore vacuum drain as the abdominal wall was rather fat.

86 The completed operative field showing the skin closed with a continuous subcuticular absorbable suture, the wound drained with a vacuum drain and the stomach drained by a gastrostomy.

87

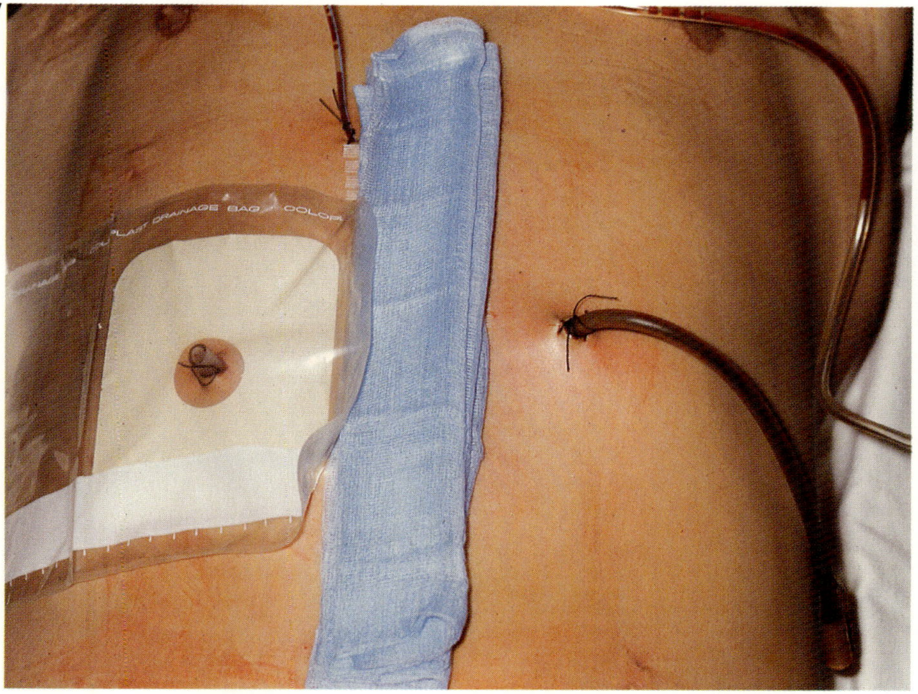

87 At the end of the operation the drainage tube is sutured to the skin and empties into an adherent plastic bag to monitor the quantity and quality of the drained fluid. The main wound is closed and the vacuum drain to the subcutaneous space is connected to a vacuum pump or vacuum bottle. The gastrostomy wound is sprayed with a plastic spray.

88

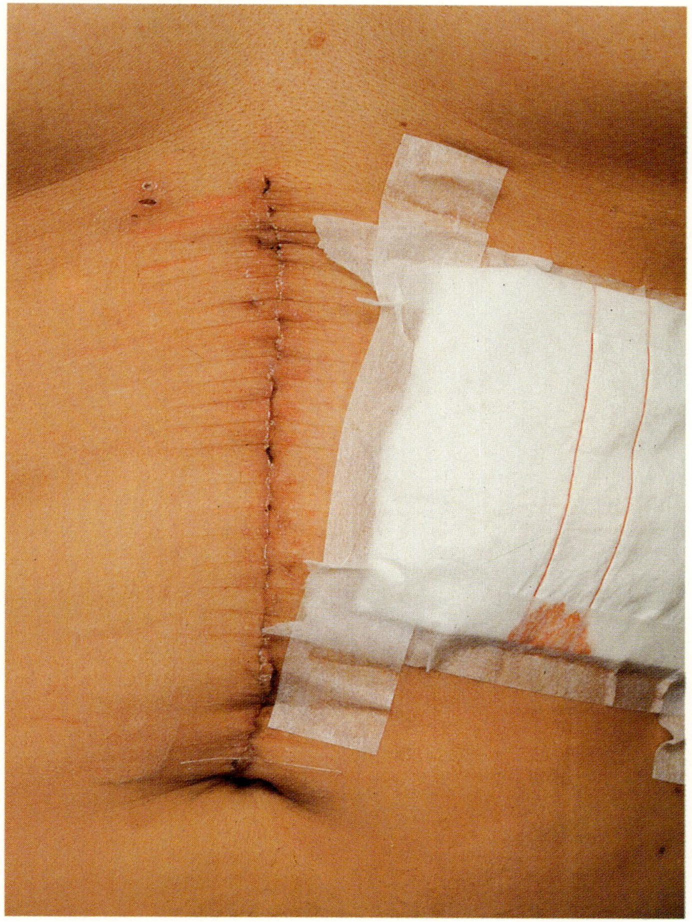

88 After about 9 to 10 days the gastrostomy tube is removed and the wound covered with a pad. The gastrostomy drainage usually stops within 24 hours of the tube being removed.

89

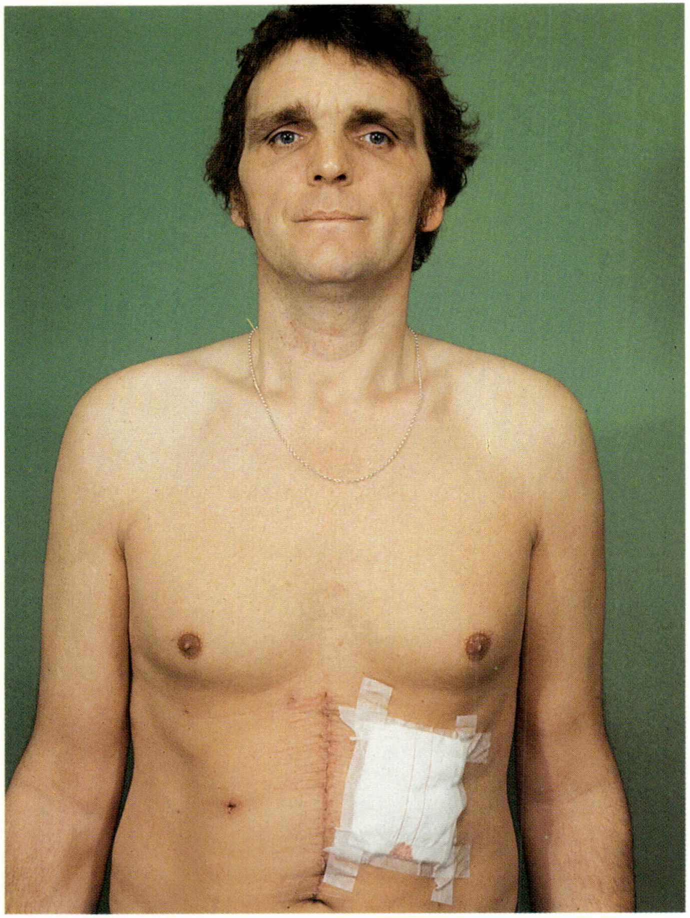

89 The patient, who is beginning to eat a light diet, is now ready to leave hospital. Most patients stay in for between 10 and 14 days after the operation.

Postoperative management

Intravenous fluid and electrolyte infusion is continued through a peripheral vein until adequate oral fluid intake is well established. It is worth considering changing the peripheral vein site for infusion every three days to reduce the risk of thrombophlebitis.

The nasogastric tube, when this is used, is maintained until the cumulative 24-hour fluid aspirate is 250ml less than the fluid intake. **It is essential to keep accurate intake and output charts.** The gastrostomy tube, which is often used instead of nasogastric intubation, is similarly left on free drainage until the output is 250ml per day less than the input. The tube is then clamped. The gastrostomy tube is not removed from the stomach until at least the eighth postoperative day. Then, the skin suture is divided and the inflation of the balloon catheter cut with scissors to allow the fluid to escape. The tube is then removed and a small dressing applied over the gastrostomy site. This is usually only necessary for 48 hours. Discharge through the gastrostomy usually stops within an hour or two of removing the tube.

The patient is allowed to have clear fluids by mouth while the stomach is undergoing tube drainage. I usually start by allowing the patient 50ml an hour and rapidly increase it to 100ml an hour to improve morale. Feeding is not usually begun until there is clear evidence of satisfactory gastric emptying of fluids and until after the bowels have been moved.

After gastric reconstruction operations in particular feeding should progress very slowly, remaining for some time on very small and semi-solid food. Large particles and dry food may be slow to empty from the stomach initially and are best avoided for some weeks.

With an uninterrupted recovery the patient can usually go home on the ninth or tenth postoperative day. Postoperative review is usually arranged at one, three and 12 months.

Antibiotic prophylaxis against aerobic and anaerobic bacteria is always given for 24-hours. As the risk of infection is so high after this operation I believe that there is a case to be made for five-day prophylaxis. I do not prescribe anticoagulants for this operation because of the risk of internal bleeding from the division of adhesions particularly under the liver. I prefer to employ antiembolus compression stockings which are worn day and night until the patient is ready to leave hospital. Ambulation is begun as early as possible.

Early postoperative complications

These can either be general or specific for the operation. General complications such as infection of the chest, the urinary system or the wound are similar to those expected for patients of this age group who may be debilitated. **Wound infection is a particularly common problem and if I feel the risk is particularly high, I leave the skin unsutured to heal by granulation.**

Infection around the gastrostomy site is particularly common, the irritation of the latex of the gastrostomy tube often predisposes to a superficial infection and this begins to cause the patient some discomfort after the fifth or sixth postoperative day. However it is rarely a major problem.

Early complications specific to this particular operation include intra-abdominal collections of blood or bile, particularly from dissection around the liver. These may become infected and lead to a sub-heptatic or sub-phrenic abscess. This complication should always be suspected in a patient who is not doing well. If confirmatory signs such as pyrexia or leucocytosis occur, the patient is monitored by ultrasound scanning or with needle exploration if indicated.

Leakage from one or other of the suture lines is the most serious complication and fortunately occurs only rarely. It is most likely to occur in severely malnourished patients or those presenting particular technical difficulties such as dense adhesions. Sometimes when adhesions of small bowel have been particularly difficult to divide, inadvertent damage to the small bowel can occur. In all cases where dissection has been very difficult I employ the air or carbon dioxide inflation technique of blowing up the loops of bowel under tension and milking the air bolus through the bowel to ensure that there is no gas leakage.

The commonest early complication is delayed emptying of the gastric remnant. This occurs frequently and is best prevented by the slow introduction of feeding. The Roux-en-Y operation usually causes a temporary disturbance of the motility of the afferent jejunal loop; I believe that it is motility dysfunction rather than anastomotic stenosis that is the principal cause of delayed emptying. If delayed emptying is suspected it can be assessed radiologically which may show also a food bezoar in the gastric remnant. **Endoscopy is the most important investigation of a patient to exclude organic obstruction;** I believe that this procedure can be usually performed safely after the tenth postoperative day. Bolus or bezoar obstruction is best dealt with by attempts at enzymatic breakdown of the bolus. This may be accompanied, if necessary, by mechanical suction through a wide bore tube. We have found that metacopramide is usually inaffective in affecting the speed of recovery from this complication.

Late complications include what I call the "four dreaded D's", dysphagia, dyspepsia, dumping and diarrhoea.

Dysphagia is usually transient, due to the trauma of dissection around the oesophagus, particularly during a revagotomy. It almost invariably subsides spontaneously.

Dyspepsia or continued food related discomfort is common after gastric reconstruction operation and frequently undermines the morale of the patient who has gone through what is often a long saga of operations and reoperations. As soon as the patient begins to experience other untoward systems they soon become depressed. For this reason **it is important to warn the patient that they may have transient indigestion.** I believe that this can be due to a variety of causes; principally delayed gastric emptying. Occasionally it is accompanied by nausea and vomiting.

Dumping sometimes recurs as soon as the efferent jejunal loop starts to empty normally and is particularly common after fluids ingestion. The patients are warned that they might experience dumping and are told that the symptom will usually have disappeared by six to 12 months. Patients who suffer from it are advised to take small, dry frequent meals and if possible to lie down after a big meal, particularly in the early months after operation.

Diarrhoea may occur but appears to be less common after gastric reconstruction operations than after the, apparently smaller, operations of vagotomy and pyloroplasty. It is related largely to the speed of gastric emptying. It is usually best controlled by simple anti-diarrhoeal agents and tend to become less severe with time.

Recurrent or stomal ulceration rarely occurs, if there has been an adequate vagotomy of the gastric remnant. If recurrent ulcer is demonstrated endoscopically after gastric reconstruction with adequate vagotomy, one should suspect retained antrum tissue attached to the duodenal stump and serum gastric levels should be measured.

Index

All figures refer to page numbers